To be returned on or before
the last date stamped below

NORTHERN COLLEGE
LIBRARY RESOURCE CENTRE

Gardyne Road, Broughty Ferry, Dundee DD5 1NY
Telephone 01382 464267

The borrower is personally responsible for this Library material.
Any transfer to another person must be done through the Library.

198

HEALTH AND LIFESTYLES

HEALTH AND LIFESTYLES

MILDRED BLAXTER

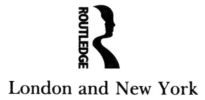

London and New York

First published 1990
by Routledge
11 New Fetter Lane, London EC4P 4EE

Simultaneously published in the USA and Canada
by Routledge
29 West 35th Street, New York, NY 10001

Reprinted 1992, 1993, 1995

© 1990 Mildred Blaxter

Typeset in Garamond by
J&L Composition Ltd, Filey, North Yorkshire
Printed and bound in Great Britain by
Mackays of Chatham PLC, Chatham, Kent

A Tavistock/Routledge Publication

British Library Cataloguing in Publication Data
A catalogue record for this book is available from the British Library

Library of Congress Cataloguing in Publication Data
A catalogue record for this book is available from the Library of
Congress

ISBN 0-415-00146-3 (hbk)   ISBN 0-415-00147-1 (pbk)

CONTENTS

CONTENTS

LIST OF FIGURES

LIST OF FIGURES

ACKNOWLEDGEMENTS

The Health and Lifestyle Survey, which provided the data for this volume, was conducted by a multi-disciplinary team under Dr B.D. Cox at the Office of the Regius Professor of Physic and the Department of Psychiatry, University of Cambridge School of Clinical Medicine. Fieldwork was carried out by Social and Community Planning Research. The survey was funded by the Health Promotion Research Trust, to whom grateful acknowledgement is due not only for their initiative in promoting the study but also for my support during the period of this analysis. The views expressed in this volume are of course mine and not those of the Trust.

A major debt is owed to Judith Nickson, who not only acted as data manager for the survey, but also gave invaluable assistance during the preparation of this volume. Acknowledgement is also due to individual members of the original team, whose work in designing and analysing particular sections of the survey has been drawn upon: Brian D. Cox (physiological measurements), Felicia A. Huppert (psychological measures), Margaret J. Whichelow (diet and smoking), Nigel Fenner (exercise and leisure), and Jean Stark (social contacts). Thanks are also owed to Lesley Davies for her very willing help in the preparation of this volume.

Chapter One

INTRODUCTION

At the individual level, ill health may often seem to strike randomly. At the level of populations, however, it is well known that circumstances and ways of living are closely associated with health: poverty or prosperity, an urban or a rural environment, work and unemployment, stress and contentment – all these have an influence upon health. What fosters a 'healthy' lifestyle? How much responsibility does the individual have for his or her own health? These questions are currently at the forefront of public attention. Certain behaviour patterns are thought to be crucially related to the major diseases which are now prominent in advanced societies. More generally, interest has grown in the positive aspects of health and in health promotion. This movement is tied to rising public expectations of better health (WHO 1984). The ways in which the different factors which influence health interact are complex, however, and the relative importance of different aspects of life is not easy to gauge.

In 1984/5 a large national survey of the population of England, Wales and Scotland, the Health and Lifestyle Survey, was carried out. In it, people were asked in great detail about their health and their lifestyles, certain aspects of their fitness were measured, and they were invited to express their opinions and attitudes towards health and health-related behaviour. Because so many aspects of life are included about the same individuals, the opportunity arises to look in a very general way at the relationship between attitudes, circumstances, behaviour and health.

This volume attempts, first, to assess what 'health' means to people, and how it is distributed in the population. Then, the questions are asked: how do health-related behaviour and less 'voluntary' aspects of social circumstances interact, and which is the more important? To what extent is 'inequality' in health the failure of individuals to take responsibility for their health, and to what extent the result of environments which induce vulnerability? How much of 'healthy' behaviour is purposive, and based on accurate beliefs and positive attitudes to health promotion, and what are the factors which facilitate or prevent healthy lifestyles?

To suggest that definitive answers could be given to these questions is certainly over-ambitious. This analysis is no more than descriptive and model-building, and in modelling one is to some extent creating an artificial world, in which the infinite variety of human lives is glossed over. However, the study of the general determinants of health has been neglected in Britain, except for small-scale studies, or research on particular diseases (such as heart disease), or the study of particular health-related habits (such as smoking). We have nothing to compare, for instance, with the work of the Human Population Laboratory in the United States (Berkman and Breslow 1983) where the influence of lifestyle factors on health has been studied for over twenty years. The Health and Lifestyle Survey suffers from the great disadvantage, in comparison, of having no longitudinal element, so that any statements about cause and effect must be very tentative. The analysis presented here is, however, offered as a first attempt to consider the lives of individuals as a whole, with all the varied influences which bear upon their health.

Health

First, 'health' must be defined. There are no simple or obvious ways in which this can be done, as a great deal of literature over the past twenty or thirty years testifies (e.g. National Center for Health Statistics 1964; Belloc *et al.* 1971; Breslow 1972; Elinson 1974; Balinsky and Berger 1975; Chen and Bryant 1975; Kaplan *et al.* 1976; Sackett *et al.* 1977; Stacey 1977; WHO 1979; Ware *et al.* 1981; Headey *et al.* 1985; Kirshner and Guyatt 1985).

Disease or physiological status can be identified or measured (though less easily in a large population survey), but this is not the whole of health: health and illness are social as well as biological facts. Lay people themselves are very aware of this, as the data on concepts of health in Chapter 3 will show. The way in which the respondents to the survey defined the concept of health is dealt with in this early chapter because it seems important, in a survey in which people are asked to talk about health, to bear in mind what they appear to mean by it.

In the biomedical model on which much of modern medicine is based, disease is defined as deviations of measurable biological variables from the norm, or the presence of defined and categorized forms of pathology. This is certainly one component of lay models of health and illness, too. However, as many historians and philosophers of medicine have pointed out, even this apparently clear-cut view of ill health is not without its problems: the definition and classification of disease is inevitably to some extent socially constructed, and 'normality' itself is a relative and judgemental concept (Dubos 1961; Engel 1977; Ryle 1961; Mishler 1981).

The respondents to this survey demonstrated clearly that 'health', more widely defined, was for them essentially a relative state, influenced notably by the normal ageing process. Health could be identified simply as the absence of disease, but for most people it was more than that. They tended to agree, it would seem, with the World Health Organization's definition of health as a 'state of complete physical, social and mental well being and not merely the absence of disease or infirmity'.

Such broad definitions of health are not new, of course: they echo the classical Platonic model of health as harmony among the body's processes, or the Galenian concept of disease as disturbance of equilibrium. Nor are they at odds with modern scientific theories of vulnerability and immunity. Trying to operationalize such a wide concept of health has the danger of subsuming all human life and happiness under this label: nevertheless, it does draw attention to the fact that positive aspects of healthiness ought to be considered, and not only the negative aspects of pathology. It may be that it is as important to distinguish the factors which differentiate health which is above average and that which is merely average, as it is to look at those which cause the average to become 'bad'. We know much less

3

about the things which favour positive health than about those which cause disease (Brown 1981).

The definition of health used in this study, therefore, is essentially multi-dimensional and relative. It includes both objective and subjective components, and attempts to consider the positive as well as the negative range.

The search for causes

During the nineteenth century the work of Pasteur and Koch, demonstrating that specific diseases could be caused by the invasion of specific micro-organisms, gave rise to what Dubos (1961) has named the 'doctrine of specific etiology'. Illness is postulated as consisting of distinct and discrete clinical states, each with specific pathological manifestations and each caused by a different agent (Koch 1890). The subsequent era of classical epidemiology focused, with great success, upon diseases – whether caused by micro-organisms, viruses, nutrient deficiencies, toxins or other causative agents – where the model of a specific agent, giving rise to a distinct pathology, seemed appropriate.

The traditional approaches of epidemiology become more complex, however, in the modern Western world, where many of the health problems are degenerative and chronic. There is now recognition that most diseases have multiple and interactive causes. Indeed, perhaps all ill health must be viewed in this way, given modern knowledge about susceptibility, about genetic dispositions, and about the influence of psycho-social factors. More complex – if at the same time less precise and demonstrable – levels of explanation may be required.

It must be made clear that the present study does not address the classical epidemiological issues – what are the causes of specific diseases? A household survey is certainly not the most appropriate method for such questions: no study in the community can provide accurate prevalences of more serious disease, since those who are suffering from such diseases are likely to be in hospital, or at the least less likely to be available for interview. Instead of narrowing down to particular causes and particular pathologies, the intention is to build up, at the most general level possible, models of the relationship between life-style and health.

Lifestyle

'Lifestyle' is a vague term. Although it is a popular concept, what we mean by it has been questioned (McQueen 1988; Wiley and Comacho 1980; Taylor and Ford 1981). Often it is used to mean only voluntary lifestyles, the choices that people make about their behaviour and especially about their consumption patterns. In the context of health, choices about food, about smoking and drinking, and about the way in which leisure time is spent, are often thought to be the most relevant. Styles of living also have economic and cultural dimensions, however: the way of life of the city may inevitably be different from that of the country, the single from the married, the North from the South. There is overwhelming evidence for persistent socio-economic influences upon health: income, work, housing, and the physical and social environments are also part of ways of living. These have to be considered both as having a direct effect on health and as factors influencing behaviour.

This wide definition of lifestyle is the one which is used here, rather than one based on personal behaviours which are known to be risk factors. The issue of responsibility for these personal behaviours, and more generally for the maintenance of health, is of course a controversial one which has become of increasing importance. Debate has focused on whether policies aimed at health promotion should be individualistic, placing responsibility firmly on the individual and the family, or whether they should be collectivist. On the one hand, it is argued that many of the currently most important diseases are 'self-inflicted', and remedies lie in the hands of the public. On the other, it is suggested that this approach minimizes the social and economic factors which are outside the individual's control. The issue of personal liberty may be invoked in the first case: the right of individuals to do what they wish with their own lives, guided only by education about the 'right' decisions. In the second, the inability of many people to exert control over their environment and ways of living is emphasized.

This debate is a major focus of this analysis. There is no doubt that social and economic circumstances, and the more voluntary aspects of lifestyle, are both associated with health. Can evidence be offered as to which is the more important?

Inequalities in health

The issue of social inequalities in health is thus a major topic. In this context, 'inequalities' does not mean simply that individuals differ – variation in health and strength is, after all, part of the human condition – but that the differences are socially patterned, and are felt by society to be inequitable or perhaps avoidable. Concern about this sort of inequality is not, of course, new: the pioneers of public health drew attention to the social and physical environment as a primary cause of the unequal distribution of disease and death over a century ago. Chadwick, for instance, carefully recorded in 1842 that while the expectation of life of 'Gentlemen, and persons engaged in professions, and their families' in the district of Bethnal Green was only 45 years, 'Mechanics, servants, and labourers, and their families' had an average age of death of 16.

Despite the remarkable achievements in public health and disease prevention in the hundred years which followed, concern about health inequality persisted in the mid-twentieth century and was offered as a major justification for the setting up of the National Health Service in 1948. The substantive area of concern in the 1950s and 1960s was, particularly, the health and growth of children. However, remarkable decreases in infant and child mortality were achieved in the decade or two after 1940, as infections were conquered and widespread gross deprivation disappeared, and differences between social classes in child health lessened. Inequality in health as a more general issue became again a matter of public discussion only in the 1970s, leading to the publication of the Black Report in 1980. This 'rediscovery' of inequality was perhaps based on two concerns: one was the growing realization of a failure in Britain to match the absolute improvements achieved in other developed countries, and the other the suggestion that relative differences between groups of the population might not, as anticipated, be decreasing. Much discussion and research during the 1980s has reached a generally-agreed conclusion that 'It is now possible to say, without risk of serious challenge, that the differences in life expectancy associated with socio-economic position ... have been increasing since 1951' (Wilkinson 1986a:19).

This debate has related to, and largely been based on, mortality

6

rates. However, the general increase in life expectancy (principally due to the control of fatal communicable diseases and the reduction of infant deaths) has meant mortality rates which are generally low, before old age, and thus not always clearly discriminatory. Inequalities in health may not be the same as inequalities in death. A general lack of morbidity data, together with the problems of measuring 'health', means that the relationship of death rates to general health status during a lifetime is difficult to study. There has been some suggestion that morbidity differences between social classes or income groups are less marked than mortality differences, i.e. that the disadvantaged may die earlier, because of a greater prevalence of life-threatening disease, but do not necessarily suffer more 'everyday' illness. On the other hand, there is evidence (for instance, from the General Household Survey) that social class trends in the experience of chronic illness, or in the proportion of people who assess their own health as 'poor', are steeper than class differences in mortality. This is one of the major issues which the Health and Lifestyle data can address: class differences not so much in severe or life-threatening disease, as in the everyday experience of illness, in physiological fitness, and in psycho-social health.

The Black Report, and the subsequent research and discussion, have identified several alternative reasons why social class is linked to health and illness experience. There may be a direct link: the less favourable working and living conditions of those in the lowest occupational classes expose them to greater health hazards; poverty – more likely among those in lower social classes – may mean inadequate diets or poor, damp housing. There is also an increasing emphasis on the possibility of indirect links through the role of stress. The second type of explanation gives more importance to health attitudes and health-related behaviour. Riskier behaviour (smoking, unwise diets) is associated with less education and poorer circumstances. Cultural explanations such as a lack of 'future orientation', a lower valuation placed on health, or a lack of a feeling of control over health have all been suggested. The structural and the cultural or behavioural types of explanation meet when it is suggested that it is powerlessness or constraints upon resources (time, money, social skills, energy) that limit the extent to which behaviour can be a matter of choice (Graham 1984).

The Health and Lifestyle Survey can offer only a limited contribution to this debate. In particular, the 'selection' question – crudely, the extent to which people fall into, or remain in, disadvantaged circumstances because their health is poor, or the extent to which their health is a consequence of their circumstances – cannot be answered in a single cross-sectional survey. To explore these social mechanisms properly, lifelong and perhaps intergenerational studies are required (see e.g. Wadsworth 1986).

However, some investigation can be made of the apparent relative weights of economic, cultural and behavioural factors. The question is important, because it has obvious implications for policy directed at the 'cure' of inequality, or indeed attempts to improve the health of the nation in general. If ill health is seen as largely 'self-inflicted', then education, persuasion, and an emphasis on self-responsibility will be the favoured answers; if it is principally outside the individual's control, then social policy issues will be paramount. A subsidiary question which is relevant, and is particularly addressed in this survey, is the extent to which people themselves hold the individualistic or the collectivist orientations. What do they think are the determinants of health and illness?

Chapter Two

THE HEALTH AND LIFESTYLE SURVEY

The Health and Lifestyle Survey was a national sample survey of men and women, of 18 years and over, living in private households in England, Wales and Scotland. Interviewing was carried out in three waves between autumn 1984 and summer 1985, with each region of the country represented in at least two waves in order to ensure that different times of year were represented in each area.

The achieved sample size was 9,003. A selection of addresses was made randomly from electoral registers using a three-stage design, and a response rate of 73.5 per cent was achieved. Refusals accounted for 19.1 per cent of the non-response and failure to contact or other reasons for 7.4 per cent.

Information was collected at two home visits. At the first, lasting approximately one hour, an interviewer used a part pre-coded, part open-ended, schedule to elicit information on personal and family circumstances, self-reported health, health attitudes and beliefs, and health-related behaviour, with detailed questioning on four particular aspects of lifestyle: diet, exercise, smoking and alcohol consumption.

A second visit was made by a nurse, who carried out a limited range of simple physiological measurements (height, weight, girth, blood pressure, pulse rate, respiratory function and environmental and exhaled carbon monoxide). The nurse introduced the respondents to a self-completion questionnaire which assessed personality and psychiatric status, and this was later returned by post.

Because of inevitable losses from the sample at each stage, the three parts of the study necessarily produced samples of differing sizes. Of those interviewed, 82.4 per cent were measured, and 88.6 per cent of those measured returned the psychological schedule. The numbers of people of different ages, at each stage, are shown in Table 2.1. In the following chapters, where the total sample is being considered the numbers available are those which are given in this table for the interviewed population, unless otherwise noted, or, if physiological fitness is involved, the numbers given for the 'measured' population. There may be small variations, however, due to non-response to specific questions.

Table 2.1 Numbers of respondents in the Health and Lifestyle Survey

	Males			Females			Total
	Age 18–39	40–59	60+	Age 18–39	40–59	60+	
Interview survey	1,668	1,240	997	2,150	1,596	1,352	9,003
Measurements made by nurse	1,429	1,074	818	1,810	1,311	972	7,414
Psychological schedule completed	1,126	943	745	1,625	1,174	859	6,572

The study population was compared with the 1981 Census, in order to demonstrate whether or not it could be assumed to represent accurately the population of England, Wales and Scotland. The Survey has a slight excess of women, at most ages, but some short-fall among both women and men aged 18–20, and among very elderly women. These are, of course, likely to be due to differences in availability for interview. Comparison with the Census and other national data on characteristics such as employment status, social class, marital status, household composition, etc., suggest that the study appears to offer a good and representative sample of the population, though those with the least education and lowest income were a little less likely to complete all three stages of the study.

Strengths and limitations of the data

The major feature of this very large data bank, for the purpose of this analysis, is the wide variety of types of information available about each individual. Health was enquired about in many different ways – symptoms and everyday complaints, diseases (whether or not medically diagnosed) and their consequences in the individual's daily life, prescription and non-prescription drugs being taken, and conditions suffered in the past. To set beside this account of self-reported health there is, uniquely on so large a population, some objective evaluation of fitness. There are also measures of psychological status (on a high proportion of the sample) and accounts of feelings of social support or isolation, stress and worry, well-being or malaise. Thus there are many different items of information available to contribute to a definition of health.

This may be set beside family and working circumstances, education and income, social activities and social networks, and detailed information on the four 'behaviours' studied. In addition, there is extensive data on health attitudes and beliefs – in relation to the individual's own life, about specific diseases and their causes, and more generally about health as a concept. A large-scale survey such as this is not perhaps the best method of eliciting attitudes and beliefs, which are more usually studied on a smaller scale and by more intensive methods. However, attempts were made in several ways to avoid the limitations of the structured questionnaire method. A high proportion of the questions, throughout the interview, were specifically designed to be analysed not as individual items of information – as such, they might have little validity on their own – but as part of indices which represent general orientations and beliefs expressed in different contexts. As many of the questions as possible were also open-ended, with the respondents invited to reply in their own words. Thus the problems of forced-choice answers or an imposed vocabulary may have been avoided, though (as discussed in Chapter 7) the difficulty will always remain of judging whether people are merely giving the answers they think are expected of them.

In short, there appears to be enough data, however imperfect, to attempt a classification, at the level of individuals, of some of the relationships between behaviour, circumstances, attitudes, and health.

A major limitation, however, already mentioned in Chapter 1, is the fact that this is only cross-sectional information. The

11

analysis must not make claims heavier than the data can bear, nor be regarded as 'proving' cause and effect in the complicated relationships examined. Moreover, the high level of abstraction necessary for the examination of broad models (for instance the assignment to people of characteristics such as 'in good health', 'socially isolated', 'with a positive attitude to health', 'rural dweller', and so on) means that the individual is inevitably crudely categorized.

Other important limitations include the fact that not every area of life, or everything that people can do, which is relevant to health is studied. As noted in Chapter 6, a wide range of potentially relevant health-promoting or illness-preventing actions are omitted, and the survey has no information on the use of health services.

Presentation of the analysis

For the most part, the variables used in this analysis are at best ordinal: that is, they are categories, even if ranked, rather than continuous measures. Thus only non-parametric statistics are appropriate. The sophisticated methods of statistical analysis which are nowadays available are used only sparingly: there is a progression from the use of simple proportions and ratios, to more complex methods as the analysis proceeds. The emphasis is on the individual, the single person with all his or her complicated patterns of circumstances. For this purpose, multi-variate analysis may conceal more than it illuminates: its use is therefore largely reserved until these patterns have been fully explored. It may also be noted that statistical tests of 'significance' are used only rarely. The principal method employed to measure health – standardized ratios – does not make the use of significance tests appropriate: these statistics must be regarded only as descriptive.

What is presented in the following chapters is a picture, at one moment of time, of the health of the population and what appear to be the major influences upon it. The picture is over-simplified, but by the same token is perhaps less susceptible to becoming out of date as details of circumstances and behaviour within society change. It may be that some essentially un-changing relationships can be demonstrated.

Chapter Three

WHAT IS HEALTH?

What do people mean when they talk of 'health'? Since part of this analysis concerns people's attitudes to health, their ideas about the causes of illness, and the relationship between attitudes and behaviour, it is necessary to consider whether different people are thinking of health in entirely different ways. Clearly, concepts of health will affect ideas about responsibility.

Some researchers have gone so far as to suggest that, since health is essentially subjective, the only valid measure to accept is people's own assessment of whether they are healthy or not. There are, however, problems in adopting this approach, especially if we do not know what the respondents have in mind when they use the word 'health'. Standards vary among different social groups and depend very much on age and experience: self-assessments can be very individual and eccentric. Nevertheless, the outcome measures which are used in the analysis of a population survey ought at least to take some account of what health means to lay people.

As noted in Chapter 1, a dichotomy has traditionally been seen between the biomedical or scientific model of health and a looser, more holistic model. These are sometimes falsely regarded as 'medical' and 'non-medical' ways of looking at health. Crudely, medical knowledge is seen as based on universal, generalizable science, and lay knowledge as unscientific, based on folk knowledge or individual experience. The lay concepts discussed in this chapter are not, however, being presented as necessarily or essentially different from medical concepts. In western societies, an intermixing is inevitable: lay people have been taught to think, at least in part, in biomedical

13

terms. Nor is modern medicine entirely wedded, in practice, to a narrowly-defined biomedical science: holistic concepts are also part of medical philosophy. The lay concepts which were expressed in this survey are, of course, sometimes less informed or expert than those of medical professionals. In other ways, however – since health must in part be subjectively experienced – they may be better informed. As other studies have found, they are often complex, subtle, and sophisticated.

Previous studies of lay concepts

Lay concepts of health, among 'ordinary' people in western industrialized societies, have been seen as an interesting subject of research only during the past 15 years or so. Most studies have been relatively small in scale. Perhaps the most notable was one of the first: Herzlich's (1973) study of a sample of individuals, predominantly middle class, from Paris and Normandy. These respondents distinguished clearly between illness – the negative concept – which was produced by ways of life and especially urban life, and the positive concept of health, which came from within. Health was identified as having three dimensions: the simple absence of disease, a 'reserve' of health determined by temperament and constitution, and a positive state of well-being or 'equilibrium'.

Other studies, such as those of Pill and Stott (1982) among working-class mothers of young children in South Wales, Blaxter and Paterson (1982) among two generations of Scottish working-class women, Williams (1983) among elderly people in Scotland, or Blaxter (1985) among the patients of one general medical practice, have found rather similar distinctions. Health can be defined negatively, as the absence of illness, functionally, as the ability to cope with everyday activities, or positively, as fitness and well-being. It has also been noted that in the modern world, health still has a moral dimension. Ill health and moral wrongdoing can be connected, as much among industrialized and urban populations as among primitive societies: one has a duty to be healthy, and unhealthiness implies an element of failure. Health can be seen in terms of will-power, self-discipline and self-control (Blaxter 1983).

One problem about studies such as these is that they have

concentrated on particular social groups, and it is difficult to know how generalizable the beliefs may be. Nevertheless, there have been several areas of agreement. The definition of health as positive fitness has been found to be more characteristic of those with better education or in more fortunate circumstances. In one large sample, in France, d'Houtard and Field (1984) found responses clearly linked to socio-economic class. The middle-class respondents were more likely to conceive of health in positive and expressive terms, the working class in negative and instrumental terms. Another, smaller, study of women in England (Calnan 1987) found a less clear-cut social class difference. Working-class women did, however, more frequently use a unidimensional definition that could be described as functional – 'the ability to get through the day' – while their professional counterparts were more likely to operate with multidimensional definitions which included the absence of illness and being fit as well as activity. It must be borne in mind, as Calnan points out, that these less elaborate answers of those with poorer education may be a product of the interview or survey situation, and cannot necessarily be presumed to represent differences in fundamental ideas. It has been shown in intensive, small-scale studies (Cornwell 1984, Blaxter 1983) that poorly-educated respondents, given time, can express very complex ideas on this topic. They do not always have them ready and fluent in a more superficial survey, however, and this may be relevant to the Health and Lifestyle Survey.

It is a general finding that, whatever their social class or education, people cannot always be expected to be consistent. It is very possible, as Williams (1983) has shown, to entertain two systems of thought on health-related topics at the same time, although they are at some point contradictory. These contradictions may be recognized by the informant, and elaborate attempts made to reconcile them.

Certainly, it is possible to define health as co-existing with quite severe disease or incapacity. Expressions of this from interview studies include, for instance, a Scottish woman who said of her husband that 'he had a lung taken out, but he was aye healthy enough', (Blaxter and Paterson 1982:28). Similarly, in another study, a daughter reported that her mother 'had been an active woman before this with no previous restriction apart

15

from general old age, deafness, loss of sight in one eye and loss of memory. The doctor said at the inquest she was a very fit woman for her age.' (Cartwright *et al*. 1973:41). Health or fitness have, in the minds of lay people, several different dimensions.

Alongside the three 'states' of health commonly identified – freedom from illness, ability to function, and fitness – the idea of health as 'reserve' has been found to be very prevalent. This reserve – like an economist's 'stock' of capital – can be diminished by self-neglect and accumulated by healthy behaviour. It is largely determined by heredity, influenced by childhood and traumatic events. Once spent, it leaves generalized weakness or vulnerability (Herzlich 1973; Pill and Scott 1982; Blaxter 1983). It can be exhausted, a state described by Williams' elderly respondents as being 'done, broken down, finished, cracked up, washed out', with some implication of irreversibility. Thus 'good' health is the power of overcoming disease, even if that disease is actually present: 'bad' health is being at risk, the loss of resistence even if disease is absent.

Questions used in the Health and Lifestyle Survey

It cannot be hoped that the detail and depth of studies such as these can be matched in so large a survey. Nevertheless, the opportunity does arise to test out some of these findings on a population sample.

The concepts of health discussed in this chapter are derived from answers to two questions: (1) Think of someone you know who is very healthy. Who are you thinking of? How old are they? What makes you call them healthy? (2) At times people are healthier than at other times. What is it like when you are healthy? These questions were asked at the beginning of the interview, before people had been invited to consider various aspects of health, and were presented in an open-ended way, with the respondents replying in their own words. The replies – sometimes quite long and thoughtful – were written down verbatim.

Other questions within the survey are of course relevant. Beliefs about the causes of disease, ideas about the healthiness or otherwise of lifestyles, feelings of guilt, responsibility and control – all these say something about how health is perceived.

16

These are perhaps more properly called attitudes to health, however, and discussion of them is reserved for Chapter 7. Here, it is simply the abstract concept of health which is being considered. It can be noted, however, that one of the questions used directed the respondents' minds towards other people – how does one recognize health, objectively? – and the other invited them to consider health in themselves – how does one recognize the experience of health, subjectively? It was only to be expected that rather different kinds of answer might be given. In particular, the invitation to define an abstract concept – what is it to be healthy? – provided a difficult task for many people. Many chose to interpret it in an easier way – what does it feel like to be healthy? This does not mean, however, that their answers had no value as definitions of health: a distinction can still be drawn, for instance, between those who emphasize physical states and those who stress psycho-social experience.

Broad categories of concepts of health

Tables 3.1 and 3.2 show a summary of the broad categories which were used in each context – for another, and for oneself. These are not concepts which were selected a priori, and then imposed upon the data, but categories which were derived from examination of the statements which the respondents offered. A coding frame was initially formed from a sub-sample of 100 replies, and was then checked and amplified on a further 1,000 before being applied to the whole sample. A limited number of basic concepts emerged, as shown in the tables. In general, they appear to match well with the results of other studies, except that it was clear that 'positive fitness' ought to be divided into physical fitness on the one hand, and psychological fitness on the other. These two were often mentioned together – 'to be healthy is to be physically and mentally fit' – but were clearly distinct in people's minds, since it was possible to be healthy in one sense but not the other.

Tables 3.1 and 3.2 are derived from an analysis of the replies from the total sample. Multiple answers were of course possible, and individuals cannot necessarily be assigned to a unique category. There was some tendency for better-educated respondents to offer more elaborate replies, so that in these tables

17

Table 3.1 Concepts of health used for describing someone else

	Males			Females		
	Age 18–39	40–59	60+	18–39	40–59	60+
	%					
Unable to answer, can't think of anyone, don't know why I call them healthy	10	14	23	13	12	21
Never ill, no disease	25	37	35	43	49	34
Physical fitness	44	26	10	28	20	10
Functionally able to do a lot	12	15	19	13	17	18
Psychologically fit	8	9	12	10	8	5
Leads a healthy life	22	16	11	24	16	12
In good health for age (applied to an older person)	2	8	12	3	8	15
Mean no. of concepts used by each individual offering any reply	1.3	1.3	1.2	1.4	1.4	1.2
(N = 100%)	(1,668)	(1,240)	(997)	(2,150)	(1,596)	(1,352)

Table 3.2 Concepts of health used for describing what it is to be healthy oneself

	Males			Females		
	Age 18–39	40–59	60+	18–39	40–59	60+
	%					
Unable to answer	16	12	10	11	7	8
Never ill, no disease	14	17	16	12	10	10
Physical fitness, energy	39	27	12	41	32	16
Functionally able to do a lot	22	26	43	22	36	34
Psychologically fit	31	40	36	48	52	44
Other	5	6	10	6	8	12
Mean no. of concepts used by each individual offering any reply	1.3	1.3	1.3	1.4	1.5	1.3
(N = 100%)	(1,668)	(1,240)	(997)	(2,150)	(1,596)	(1,352)

they will be represented more frequently. Subsequently in this chapter, however, the discussion and analysis is based on a random 10 per cent sample of respondents, in which it was possible to examine in a more qualitative way the precise vocabulary used and the combinations of ideas which each individual expressed. An example of the more elaborate answers to 'what is it like when you are healthy?' might be that of a 20 year-old nursing assistant in a psychiatric hospital who said:

> I feel alert and can always think of lots to do. No aches and pains – nothing wrong with me – and I can go out and jog. I suppose I have more energy, I can get up and do such a lot rather than staying in bed and cutting myself off from people.

This comprehensive definition of health includes all of the basic categories.

Each of the principal concepts identified in the more detailed analysis will be discussed in turn, looking more closely at the three classical definitions of health as absence of illness, fitness, and function. First, however, those people who found themselves unable to offer any definition of health will be considered. This is quite a large group, and it seems possible that they ought not simply to be passed over as 'non-responders'.

'Negative' answers

Almost 15 per cent of the respondents could not think of anyone who was 'very healthy', and over 10 per cent said in reply to the question about health for themselves, 'I just don't think about it', 'I can't answer that'. There is some danger in assuming that this is a negative or uninterested attitude to health, since it may indicate no more than a lack of enthusiasm about the interview situation, or a degree of inarticulacy. However, it did appear to represent a lack of thought about health, or a lack of practice in conversation about health which might have supplied a ready vocabulary. A proportion of this group, especially as Table 3.3 shows among the elderly, were expressing pessimism about their own health status: 'I'm never healthy so I don't know', 'It's so long since I was healthy that I can't tell you what it's like'.

Table 3.3 'Negative' replies to question about health for oneself

	Males			Females		
	Age 18–39	40–59	60+	18–39	40–59	60+
	%					
Can't answer because:						
I'm never healthy	2	1	3	2	3	6
Health is the norm	14	15	7	7	4	2
No elaboration	2	1	0	2	1	0
(N = 100%: 10% of sample)	(166)	(124)	(100)	(215)	(160)	(136)

However, higher proportions, especially of men under 60, were expressing the idea that health is the norm, is just 'ordinary', and so is difficult to describe:

All I know is that when I'm feeling healthy I'm not feeling ill (male technician, aged 29).

You don't realize it, you don't feel anything special until you are ill (unemployed man, aged 55).

I don't think I know when I'm healthy, I only know if I'm ill (office worker, aged 28).

How do you describe it? I don't know. I think if you are healthy you don't think about it. You only think about ill health (wife of a tractor driver, aged 51).

Though she was struggling to explain what she meant, another middle-aged woman managed to express this 'negative' definition quite clearly:

I don't really know. Sometimes I do feel less healthy, but I can't say that I feel what it is to be healthy at other times.

This group of people tended to be among those who, in other parts of the survey, did not rate health very highly as a value. They were also likely, among the elderly, to see their own health as poor. Whether old or young, they were commonly people who expressed a lack of concern for 'healthy' behaviour.

Health as not-ill

The more explicit description of health as not being ill – as not suffering any symptoms, never having anything more serious than a cold, never seeing the doctor, having no aches and pains – has also sometimes been seen as a 'negative' concept, in opposition to the positive concept of fitness. It was, as Table 3.1 showed, a more popular definition of health in another person rather than oneself, offering an easy way of 'proving' that the person was healthy:

Because he's never seen a doctor in 50 years (woman, 70, of her husband).

Someone I know who is very healthy is me, because I haven't been to a doctor yet (man of 72).

20

She's healthy because she never seems to suffer with her chest. She has an occasional cold but she's never been seriously ill (woman 70, with severe bronchitis herself, speaking of her daughter).

For oneself, more frequently than for others, 'not-ill' was expressed in terms of experienced symptoms, rather than recourse to medical services, though the nature of the symptoms naturally tended to vary with age:

Health is when you don't have a cold (man of 19).

When you don't hurt anywhere and you're not aware of any part of your body (woman of 49).

Health is when you don't feel tired and short of breath (man of 51).

You don't have to think about pain – to be free of aches and pains (woman of 78).

It has sometimes been suggested that a definition of health as 'not-ill' (or without disease) is characteristic of people in poorer circumstances, and to lack a positive view of health as fitness is a mark of general social deprivation (Blaxter and Paterson 1982). Though the latter may be true, there was little sign in this large sample of any social differentiation in the use of the concept 'not-ill': it seems possible that the previous finding may demonstrate one of the pitfalls of small-scale surveys. Because a 'negative' definition is found to be common among working-class respondents, it is assumed to be in some way associated with their social position. In fact, in this general population survey, the 'not-ill' description of health was found to be more frequently used by the better educated and those with higher incomes. It was also very markedly associated with the speaker's own state of health. At all ages, but particularly among the elderly, those who themselves were in poor health or suffering from chronic conditions were less likely to define health in terms of illness. Amongst men over 60, 22 per cent of those who were without chronic illness themselves used this definition for health in oneself, but only 10 per cent of those who did have chronic illness. The proportions among women over 60 were 16 and 6 per cent respectively. If illness symptoms are a taken for granted experience, or disease is seen as the norm, then health has to be defined in other ways.

Health as absence of disease/health despite disease

It is not always easy, in the respondent's replies, to distinguish illness – the experience of symptoms or malfunctioning – from a more clearly biomedical definition of disease. Disease was specifically mentioned rather rarely, whether for others or oneself, though phrases such as 'never had to go to hospital', 'don't have any really serious illnesses', 'never had any big illnesses', might be held to represent this concept. To have no (chronic or serious) disease is certainly one dimension of health, though not one commonly expressed by these respondents.

Certainly, however, there were expressions of a concept of health despite disease. Some 'others' were instanced who were disabled or suffering from serious conditions, yet were called healthy because they coped so well: they might be diseased but they were not ill. Many people said of themselves 'I am very healthy although I do have diabetes', or 'I am very healthy apart from this arthritis' (crippled and housebound woman of 61). The concept of health as overcoming or coping with disease could be extended to include misfortune also:

> Although he has TB he's been aware of his problems and has got over them. Though he was made redundant, since then he's done his own thing, just worked the way and when he wanted to. He didn't worry about being redundant, and he hasn't taken on too much in the size of house and garden. He enjoys life (man of 64 explaining why he calls a friend of the same age healthy).

Health as a reserve

The idea of 'healthy though diseased' often had some affinity with the 'reserve of health' noted by Herzlich. Someone is healthy because 'when he is ill he recovers very quickly', 'he has had an operation and got over it very well', or even because he takes risks and suffers no consequences: as one respondent said, 'he goes out on the drink but he never gets a hangover or a headache'. Occasionally, resondents expressed the idea of an inborn reserve of health:

He never goes to the doctors and only suffers from occasional colds. Both parents are still alive at 90 so he belongs to healthy stock (woman of 51 talking of her husband).

However, this concept was not as frequently mentioned as is usually reported in more intensive studies. It is probably an 'explanation' of health which requires more time than was available in the survey for its expression and exploration. 'Health as a reserve' was rather rarely mentioned in any explicit way for oneself, though perhaps many of the ideas which will be described as 'health as energy' do in fact come close to this concept.

Health as behaviour, health as 'the healthy life'

It can be noted in Table 3.1 that 'the healthy person' (but rarely oneself) was rather frequently defined in terms of their 'virtuous' behaviour. He or she is a vegetarian, or a non-smoker and non-drinker, or goes jogging, or does exercises:

I call her healthy because she goes jogging and she doesn't eat fried food. She walks a lot and she doesn't drink alcohol (woman of 50 about her neighbour).

She takes care of herself. She was the sickly one as a baby, but she's the healthier one now. She does all the right things. She eats plenty of fruit (woman of 64 about her daughter).

Younger people were more likely to reply briefly that the chosen 'healthy' person 'doesn't smoke or drink'. It may be that these answers are simply a way of dealing with what was seen as a difficult question: instead of attempting an answer to 'what makes you call them healthy', they were offering (rather conventional) replies to the question 'what makes them healthy'. This type of reply was strongly associated with less education and lower social class among older people, though equally likely in all classes among the young.

There is some feeling in the way this idea was expressed, however, that it was more than an evasion of the task of defining health. For these respondents, health was identical with the healthy life: the non-smoker, non-drinker must be healthy, though no evidence about their health could be offered. These respondents were also more likely to be those who, throughout the rest of the interview, stressed the role of 'bad habits' in the causation of disease and the importance of self-responsibility. As one lady said:

Why do I call her healthy? She leads a proper respectable life so she's never ill.

Health as physical fitness

Among the more positive definitions of health, whether for oneself or another, Tables 3.1 and 3.2 showed that among younger people, physical fitness was very prominent. As might be expected, it was a less favoured concept among men and women over 60. When thinking of 'the healthy person', young men in particular stressed strength, athletic prowess, the ability to play sports: 'fit' was by far the most common word used in their descriptions of health by men under 40. The 'healthy other' was, for them, likely to be either a well-known athlete or sportsman, or a personal acquaintance who ran marathons, played squash, engaged in karate or judo, or 'trained every week'. Weight-lifting and body-building were very frequently mentioned as a source of, and a proof of, fitness. Older men also mentioned sportsmen, though less frequently. Young women, too, commonly expressed a concept of health (in others) that involved sports and physical fitness.

This is one reason why the sex of the 'person thought of as healthy' was predominantly male. Among those who offered any answer, whatever concept of health they were expressing, 80 per cent of males mentioned a man, and 57 per cent of females also mentioned a man. Few women athletes appeared as role models. (Other reasons why women were less likely to be thought of as healthy will, however, be suggested.)

Health for oneself, for many young men and some older men, was also defined as physical strength and fitness:

There's a tone to my body, I feel fit (man of 24).

I can do something strenuous and don't feel that tired after I've done it (man of 26).

I can walk up the stairs to this flat, without a pause, 16 flights and I hardly use the lift, and I'm not out of breath (driver of 44).

Women rarely mentioned sports or specific physical leisure pursuits. They did, however, frequently define physical fitness in terms of its outward appearance. They commonly mentioned being (or feeling) slim. To be fit was to have a clear complexion, bright eyes and shining hair:

> Being healthy is when my skin is good and my hair isn't greasy and I can do all the things I want to without feeling tired (woman of 30).

Health as energy, vitality

The last quotation combines the notions of an appearance of fitness with a feeling of energy or vitality. 'Energy' was in fact the word most frequently used by all women and older men to describe health, and for younger men it came a close second to 'fitness'. Sometimes physical energy was clearly meant, and sometimes a psycho-social vitality which had little to do with physique: most often, the two were combined.

The words used to describe this were 'lively', 'alert', 'full of get up and go', 'full of life', 'not tired', 'not listless'. As one young man said:

> Health is when I feel I can do anything. I jump out of bed in the morning, I wash my car in the cold without a thought. I feel like doing things. Nothing can stop you in your tracks (engineer of 28).

Many young men, like this one, mentioned getting up early, or not going to bed so early at night: 'it's easier to get out of bed', 'I feel like getting up in the morning', 'I don't spend all morning in bed', 'You can afford to sleep less at night'. Even as a description of the healthy 'other', not staying in bed appeared to mark really positive healthiness:

> He regularly wakes up early in the morning, gets up, doesn't watch a lot of TV (man of 21).

For older men, the same concept of energy and vitality was most often expressed as enthusiasm about work:

> I can give myself to work a hundred per cent. Work is a pleasure. Work's not a problem (Council engineering employee, aged 49).

You feel ready to get on with anything that needs doing. You feel that you can tackle any physical work (man of 74).

Women, too, very commonly defined healthiness in terms of energy and enthusiasm for work. It was notable, however, that few of any age, whether or not they had a job outside the home, mentioned paid work. The symbol of energy for women was 'going right through the house', 'cleaning the house from top to bottom': 14 per cent of all women under 60 mentioned enthusiasm about housework. For elderly women, being *able* to do housework might be a mark of health, but for the younger, who took their everyday work for granted, *enjoyment* of housework indicated special energy. Certain less popular jobs were singled out:

I clean the windows and rush round like a mad thing. When I'm not healthy is when I want to sit in front of the box (single-handed mother, kitchen assistant, aged 29).

When I'm healthy I feel like tackling the cooker and getting it clean (female teacher, aged 47).

Particularly for women, however, the concept of 'energy' was a very positive one, not wholly captured by 'feeling like doing things' or 'not being tired'.

Health is having loads of whumph. You feel good, you look good, nothing really bothers you, everything in life is wonderful, you seem to feel like doing more (married woman, aged 28, part-time office worker).

Similarly, women of every age defined health as 'bright in mind and body', 'doing everything easily', 'feeling like conquering the world', 'being keen and interested', 'lots of get up and go', 'properly alive', 'having the energy to be with other people'.

Health as social relationships

A notable difference between men and women was that women were considerably more likely to define health, especially in themselves, in terms of their relationships with other people. Only a handful of men did so, and then usually by reference to their own moods:

When I'm healthy I'm very talkative. If I'm feeling low I keep myself to myself – I'm very outgoing when I'm well, and not moody (male shop manager, aged 22).

A few others identified health with 'not being grumpy', 'not short with people', 'you treat people better'. For women of all ages, however, health was often located within their social relationships. Approximately 8 per cent of women under 60, and 12 per cent of women over 60, mentioned their families or 'other people' in their definitions of health for themselves. Even the concept of health in others could often include their social relationships and attitudes to those around them:

I call him healthy because of his general approach to life. He's an open individual, always ready to join in (woman, aged 44 talking of her 20-year-old son).

She goes around looking after friends and shopping for them. She's active, her mind's alive. She paints and she's a member of the theatre club and a lot of other groups (woman of 51 speaking of her mother of 77).

For younger women, health was commonly defined in terms of good relationships with family and children – 'having more patience with them', 'coping with the family', 'enjoying the family'. For the older, serving other people, being in a position to help other people, having sufficient energy to care for other people, were often cited as the marks of good health. Those women who identified a female as 'someone who is very healthy' quite commonly said 'I call her healthy because she's always doing things for other people'. For health in themselves, they said 'You're more willing to meet people and help people', or 'I could do anything, help anyone'. This was a particularly frequent reply of more elderly women:

To be well in health means I feel I can do others a good turn if they need help (woman of 79, disabled with arthritis).

You feel as though everyone is your friend, I enjoy life more, and can work, and help other people (woman of 74).

Health as function

Both health as energy, and health as social relationships, are concepts which overlap with the idea of health as function –

health defined by being able to do things, with less stress upon a description of feelings. Health as function, as Tables 3.1 and 3.2 showed, was more likely to be expressed by older people: for the young, of course, the ability to cope with the tasks of life might be taken for granted, and it is only later in life that health may be seen as a generally restricting factor.

For men below retirement age, and especially those who did manual work, health for oneself or for others could be defined as being able to do hard work. Many women who identified a man (usually their husband) as 'someone who is very healthy' also gave as their reason the physically demanding nature of his work, or the fact that he was able to work long hours. Although women were chosen as a 'healthy other' because of their general social, family and community activity, it was notable that neither sex often chose women because of their demanding work, whether within the house or outside it.

However, many elderly men and women were identified as 'someone I know who is very healthy' because they were able to work despite an advanced age:

> She's 81 and she gets her work done quicker than me, and she does the garden (woman of 63).

Similarly, health for oneself in old age was frequently defined as being able to do 'extra work', or being fit to work, as well as being mobile or self-sufficient:

> Being healthy is when I walk to my work on a night, and I walk to school to collect the grandchildren (woman, aged 76, employed part-time in a woollen mill).

> Health is being able to walk around better, and doing more work in the house when my knees let me (woman of 79).

Several people, among the young as well as the elderly, expressed a concept of health as 'being able to do what you want to when you want to' – that is, a definition of health as not being restricted or hampered. Some half-dozen, of differing ages, said simply and explicitly that 'health is freedom'.

Health as psycho-social well-being

The concept of health as psycho-social well-being is often close to or combined with the notions of health as energy, health as social relationships, or health as function, which have been discussed. In the analysis shown in Tables 3.1 and 3.2, the category was reserved, however, for expressions of health as a purely mental state, instead of, or as well as, a physical condition. This is difficult to describe in another person, though as Table 3.1 showed, nearly 10 per cent of the sample used expressions such as 'mentally alert', 'happy and relaxed', or 'enjoys life', in their descriptions of 'someone who is very healthy'. Often, these were embedded in a very holistic view of health:

She's a person with a spiritual core. She's physically, mentally and spiritually at one (single woman, aged 45, living in a religious community).

For health in oneself, as Table 3.2 showed, psycho-social health was stressed at all ages, and for those in the middle years was the most popular concept. It tended to be used rather more frequently by women than by men, and by those with more education rather than less. 'Health is a state of mind' or 'health is a mental thing more than physical' were common statements. Among young men, 'confidence' and 'pride' were popular words:

Health is to feel proud – when you can go out and you can hold your head up, look good. You don't have so many hang-ups and you can think straight. You have a clear mind (male computer operator, aged 25).

For older men, the favoured expressions were 'relaxed', 'not worried', 'happy'. Women also used the words 'relaxed' and 'happy', but tended to offer more elaborate and enthusiastic descriptions than the majority of men:

Emotionally you are stable, energetic, happier, more contented and things don't bother you so. Generally it's being carefree, you look better, you get on better with other people (single woman of 20, a secretary).

I'm at peace with myself. Energetic, outgoing. I can cope with more pressures than usual, with the demands made by other people. I have the capacity to know when I've had enough, whereas if I'm less healthy, tired, I'm inclined to go on too long. When I'm bad, well, I just want to hide away (single woman, aged 48).

'Feel like living life to the full', 'on top of the world', 'full of the joys of spring', were phrases very commonly repeated. More elderly women who felt themselves to be, at least part of the time, in good health, were particularly likely to associate happiness and health, using expressions like 'happy to be alive', 'glad to get up each day', 'a joy to be living'. Their descriptions of health ranged from the simple:

> Well, I think health is when you feel happy. Because I know when I'm happy I feel quite well (woman of 72);

to the very enthusiastic:

> I've reached the stage now where I say isn't it lovely and good to be alive, seeing all the lovely leaves on the trees, it's wonderful to be alive and to be able to stand and stare! (farmer's widow, aged 74).

Concepts of health through the life course

Though these brief replies to a few questions cannot hope to match the analysis possible in more intensive studies of concepts of health, the large number of respondents does permit some firm conclusions to be offered.

Firstly, the way in which health is conceived of differs over the life course, in not unexpected ways. Younger men tend to speak of health in terms of physical strength and fitness, and commonly cite athletes as the 'healthy other'. Young women, though they also talk of fitness or its appearance, favour ideas of energy, vitality, and ability to cope. In middle age, concepts of health become more complex, with an emphasis upon total mental and physical well-being. Older people, particularly men, think in terms of function, or the ability to do things, though ideas of health as contentment, happiness, a state of mind – even in the presence of disease or disability – are also prominent.

Secondly, there are clear sex differences. At all ages women, in general, gave more expansive answers than men, and appeared to find the questions more interesting. Women of higher social class or higher educational qualifications, in particular, expressed many-dimensional concepts. Many women, but few men, included social relationships in their definition of health.

Thirdly, it is obvious that health is not a unitary concept. Ideally, it includes all possible dimensions. The 'negative' definition of health as 'not ill, no disease' has within itself at least two dimensions: the absence of symptoms, or feeling ill, and 'wholeness', or absence of diagnosed pathology. Sometimes these are clearly separate, as when a respondent defined health as being without aches and pains even though chronic disease was present.

OWN ASSESSMENT OF HEALTH

It might be expected that these individual ways of defining health would be associated with the speaker's self-assessed health status. Perhaps those who define health as physical strength and fitness judge their own health on these criteria; alternatively, perhaps one's own state of health dictates the way in which health is conceptualized. This survey, like many others, asked the respondents to assess their own health as 'excellent, good, fair or poor, compared with someone of your own age'. There have been many studies of the meaning or 'accuracy' of the replies to this question. Such a subjective measure may be dismissed as meaningless, since one does not know what standards people are using, or how their assessments may be affected by an unwillingness to label their own health as poor. On the other hand, self-defined health has been shown to be one of the better predictors of mortality (Singer *et al.* 1976) and to be important in aspects of adjustment to major illness (Hunt *et al.* 1980).

The Health and Lifestyle Survey not only offers the opportunity to examine how self-assessments relate to health measured in many different ways (a topic which will be considered later), but also to consider the relevance of different concepts of health. To ask people to define their own health in these broad categories is the simplest possible 'measure' of health status. Is it a useful one, or is it too dependent on the various ways in which people may think about health?

The patterning of self-assessed health

In this survey, as in others, the majority of respondents (71 per cent) defined their health as at least good. Good health, as the discussion of concepts has suggested, did not necessarily exclude disease or mean that the respondent was free from symptoms of illness. Indeed, many disabled and/or elderly people insisted on calling their health 'excellent', even though this seemed an optimistic definition: an example was a man of 71, with several chronic conditions, wheelchair-bound and requiring assistance with most of the activities of daily living. Obviously, these people were saying 'my health is excellent considering my advanced years', or 'my health is excellent despite my disability'. Equally obviously, however, there is a preference among the public at large for defining their own health as good if at all possible.

As found in other studies (for instance, successive editions of the General Household Survey), there were steep and regular differences in self-assessed health by all measures of social advantage or disadvantage. Those in lower classes were more likely to say that their health was only fair or poor, especially in older years. Single-handed parents, the unemployed, those living in inner cities and industrial areas, were all more likely than their peers to present a depressed view of their health. In Scotland, 31 per cent of men and 33 per cent of women said their health was less than good, compared with 23 per cent of men and 24 per cent of women in the South East (with rates standardized for the age distribution of the region).

An analysis by four arbitrarily-defined groups of high or low household income illustrated in Figure 3.1 (in which younger and older people are distinguished, since low incomes are more likely among the elderly), epitomizes and summarizes this relationship of self-defined health to social or environmental circumstances. The question remains, of course – and is, indeed one of the principal questions this volume seeks to answer – about the extent to which these are simply realistic judgements about actual health.

At the individual level, however, it is clear that there are many anomalous self-assessments. Irrespective of social circumstances, a pessimistic view of one's own health was, for instance, associated very strongly with personality characteristics such as neuroticism, as measured by the Eysenck Personality Inventory which formed part of the self-completion personality tests.

The use of the different concepts of health was also strongly associated with defining one's own health as good/excellent, or

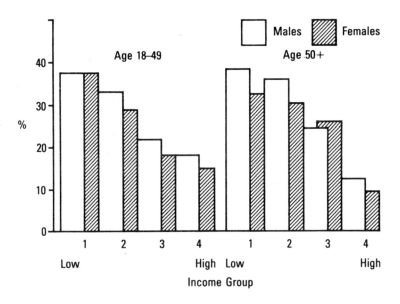

Figure 3.1 Proportions of men and women who assessed their own health as only 'fair' or 'poor', in four groups of household income

only fair/poor. As Table 3.4 shows, those who thought their own health was not good were, not unexpectedly, more likely to be in the group who were unable to offer any description of health. 'Function' as a definition of health did not appear to be related to self-defined health status. The concept of 'never ill, not diseased' was, however, more likely to be used by those who thought their own health good. Especially among men, health was also more likely to be described as 'fitness' by those who said their health was good; there is of course an association here between youth (and thus, probably, better health) and the choice of 'fitness' as a definition, but it was true at all ages that the self-defined 'healthy' were likely to favour this concept. Many who described health in terms of fitness appeared to be saying guiltily, when their replies to the self-assessment question were compared with other comments about their lives, 'I am not as fit as I should be, therefore – even if I have no illness – I am not healthy'. Similarly, women (more clearly than men) who took a

33

positive view of their own health were more likely to offer a definition of health in terms of psycho-social well-being.

Table 3.4   Own assessment of health related to concept of health used to describe health in oneself
(Per cent of those defining own health as good/excellent, or as fair/poor, who used concept, all ages)

	Males		Females	
	Defining own health as			
Concept of health	Good/ex.	Fair/poor	Good/ex.	Fair/poor
None	9	24**	5	19**
Never ill, no disease	18	9**	13	6*
Physical fitness, energy	31	21**	33	28*
Functionally able	28	29	29	32
Psychologically fit	36	34	51	40**
(N = 100%)	(2,790)	(1,120)	(3,623)	(1,470)

Difference between those defining own health good/ex., and fair/poor, by X^2: *$p<.01$; **$p<.001$

Does it appear that the ways in which health is viewed as a concept affect self-assessments of health status, or vice versa? The first determinants of the way in which health is conceptualized are the simple demographic variables of age and gender. Within this, though the direction of causation cannot be proved, it is the individual's own perceived health status which appears to determine the way in which health is described, rather than the reverse. It seems very probable that actual health status, and experience of disease, are crucial. Evidence about this can only be offered, however, after ways of measuring health have been considered.

Chapter Four

THE MEASUREMENT OF HEALTH

This chapter approaches the concept of health in a different way. If we wish to consider the relationship of behaviour or social circumstances to health, then health must be measured in some more objective way. How, in a population survey such as this, are these measures to be constructed?

The lay concepts discussed in Chapter 3 cannot altogether provide the basis for the measures to be chosen: some choice has to be made between contradictory interpretations of what health means, and a limit imposed which restricts the definition of health to something less than the whole of life satisfaction or human happiness. Lay concepts will, of course, affect consideration of the reliability or the meaning of the answers to questions from which the measures are constructed. It can also be argued that lay definitions of health should also at least be borne in mind, in choosing how to measure health: this is particularly important in any study which seeks to consider attitudes to health.

The most important conclusions to be drawn from Chapter 3 are probably the following:

1. Health is not, in the minds of most people, a unitary concept. It is multi-dimensional, and it is quite possible to have 'good' health in one respect, but 'bad' in another. Its components commonly vary together, but they do not necessarily do so: if one has a serious disease, then it is likely that one will 'feel ill', and suffer lack of general well-being, but there are many examples of people who say that they are 'healthy' despite disease. Psycho-social malaise is defined as ill health, even if the

individual's physical health is apparently good. An implication of this multi-dimensionality is that health status is unlikely to be susceptible to measurement along one linear scale.

2. It is difficult, bearing in mind these lay descriptions of health, to think in terms of a simple dichotomy between 'well' and 'ill'. Good health can be expressed simply as an absence of illness, but it is also a positive concept and one which has many degrees. The energy, happiness and sense of well-being described by many people is very much more than the simple absence of disease. The implication here is that survey measures should always, as far as possible, extend into positive health: they should not focus entirely upon degrees of illness.

3. Normal health, even 'good health', can accommodate an 'ordinary' level of symptoms or complaints. (What is considered to be ordinary, and compatible with good health, will obviously depend primarily upon age, but also on gender, on social norms, and on health experience.) To have no symptoms or complaints at all is, in fact, highly extraordinary, and could be described not just as good health but as super health. In this survey, only about one-fifth of men and one-sixth of women claimed to have experienced none, 'during the past month', of a checklist including 16 of the most common physical symptoms, and only 6 per cent of men and 4 per cent of women could be described, on all the evidence available, as being in 'perfect' health (no symptoms of physical illness, no known disease condition, an above average level of physiological fitness and a high level of psycho-social well-being). Obviously, it makes no sense to call only this small minority the healthy, though many health surveys do define good health simply by the absence of morbidity.

4. The functional consequences are obviously an important part of the definition of health for lay people: how do I know when I am ill? When I cannot perform my social roles. What is it to be healthy? To be able to do things. Thus the consequences of any disease or impairment ought to be taken into account in any measure. It is equally obvious, however, that they cannot be the sole factor to be considered, because what people are able to do, or choose to do, differs so much by characteristics of their environment, social situation, or personality.

5. Finally, the analysis of lay concepts suggests that neither subjective nor objective accounts of health are, alone, sufficient. A biomedical definition of health in terms of disease, abnormality or malfunction is, of course, part of the lay concept of health, but individuals may misinterpret, misinform, or be ignorant of their biomedical condition. On the other hand, health is also a subjective state, and individuals have information about their symptoms and their feeling states which only they can give.

A brief review of health indices

Because of the reasons sketched in Chapter 1, there has been an increasing interest in general health surveys of populations in recent decades (though less, perhaps, in Britain than in some other countries) and a proliferation of attempts to devise indices by which health may be described.

It is axiomatic that the value of an index depends on the purpose for which it is required and the audience that will make use of it. For some purposes, ill health may be defined in terms of the use of medical services. Attendances at or stays in hospital, consultations with medical practitioners, or the use of prescribed drugs, may be assumed to be measures of illness. However, there are obvious problems about measuring health by service-defined categories. The individual has first to make contact with services before his or her illness can be counted. Such measures confuse the demand for services and the supply of services, and are products of diagnostic practices, admission practices and local differences in service supply: they cannot be assumed to be measures of health. This is not to belittle their importance or interest in their own right, but their relationship to actual health status is a difficult area (Blaxter 1989).

For other purposes, it may be useful to define health simply in terms of its consequences:

> The concept of a morbidity condition ... includes only
> conditions as a result of which the person has taken one or
> more of various actions ... the restricting of usual activities,
> including going to bed, the seeking of medical advice, or the
> taking of medicine.
>
> (National Center for Health Statistics 1964)

37

Obviously, for administrative or social policy purposes, it may be important to know who is incapacitated by ill health, or who is likely to consume medical services. From this point of view, illness which has no consequences (in sociological terms, is not translated into sickness) is not of interest. Such scales may also be used for the study of the effect of treatment given to those who are ill, or the course of illnesses. One well-validated instrument, for instance, is the Sickness Impact Profile (Bergner *et al.* 1976), a 235-item questionnaire from which weighted additive scales can be derived, with judgements based on panel assessments, for 14 areas of life in which there may be functional incapacity, such as work, recreation, speech, movement, social and family relationships. Other indices which are designed for 'well' as well as 'ill' populations include the Functional State Index (Fanshel and Bush 1970) where health is viewed as a continuum on a linear scale, based on ability to carry out the activities 'appropriate to social roles', running from well-being through dissatisfaction and disability to coma and death. The second section of the Nottingham Health Profile (Hunt *et al.* 1980) is similarly concerned with the impact of illness on activities of different kinds.

'Functional' indices have become popular, not only because the behavioural manifestations of health are easier to measure (by survey methods) than health itself, but also because they represent a more social concept of health than accounts of disease. Part of the attraction lies in the fact that linear scales of dysfunction are easier to produce than linear scales of health, as a great deal of work specifically concerned with disability has demonstrated (e.g. the Activities of Daily Living measure, Katz *et al.* 1963; Garrad and Bennett 1971; the index developed by Sainsbury 1973; the Functional Limitation Profile of Patrick *et al.* 1981; see also Sullivan 1971). Many of the more generally applicable indices also have the advantage of extending into 'positive' health, rather than focusing only upon those who are ill. Inevitably, however, problems are raised because of the different ways in which individuals react to their ill health.

In contrast to functional measures, indices may rest solely on the presence or absence of disease or symptoms of pain and malfunctioning. Population health surveys in many countries, including the British General Household Survey, rely on simple categories of those who are experiencing symptoms but do not define themselves as having chronic conditions, and those who can name a 'long-standing illness or impairment' that they suffer from. Typical forms of the question eliciting chronic conditions are: 'Do you suffer from a physical infirmity, handicap or chronic illness which will continue to affect you in the future? (France, CREDOC 1982), or 'Do you have any long-standing illness, disability or infirmity? That is, anything that has troubled you over a period of time or is likely to affect you over a period of time?' (Britain, General Household Survey).

Obviously, the existence of disease or impairment must be one important component of health, whether or not it has (for the individual, or at the present time) any consequences in terms of distress or disability. The problem which arises with this measure relates, however, to the 'accuracy' of the replies. As Haberman commented:

> At one time respondents' reports of illness were regarded as an imperfect but valid substitute for a medical report .... The question of the validity of the reports evoked an awesome outpouring of research ... basically, the answer is that respondents in surveys are poor substitutes for physicians (or vice versa).
>
> (Haberman 1969:343)

This research has shown that self-reports are likely seriously to underestimate disease which is clinically identified. In the United States, where interview data have been compared with medical records (National Center for Health Statistics 1967, Kirscht 1971) Kirscht notes that 'the extent of non-correspondence is impressive'. For instance, correspondence between self-reports and medical records from an insurance plan was only 22 per cent for arthritis/rheumatism, or 62 per cent for diabetes. In one small British study (Blaxter 1985) there was complete agreement between general practitioner records and patients' accounts for only 64 per cent of individuals. 'Disagreement' with the doctors' records consisted primarily of respondents not mentioning all the conditions which appeared in records: the identification of the existence or absence of any chronic disease showed a better agreement of about 80 per cent.

As this study noted, there could be no assumption that either the self-reports or the medical records were necessarily correct.

Respondents were mistaken about their conditions or unwilling to declare them; equally, however, the records could be wrong, or diseases could exist which had never been brought for diagnosis. These are not necessarily to be rejected because not clinically legitimated: there are many cases in which self-diagnosis is acceptable. A survey can include only that disease which people believe themselves to have, but the status of self-diagnosed 'haemorrhoids', for instance, is not for this purpose any different from that which has been professionally identified.

Thus, the problems of this measure of ill health arise not because respondents may be wrong or because disease may be unknown – these are inevitable imperfections about which little can be done, if complete clinical examinations are impractical – but because we do not know what 'counts', for whom, as a disease which should be mentioned. The possibility arises that there may be systematic differences between groups in their readiness to answer, or their interpretation of a question. In particular, suspicion that the better-educated may give more informative answers raises problematic issues.

Responses have also been shown to depend on the way in which questions are asked. The more specific and detailed the questions, the more disease is reported. An alternative method is to offer a check-list of diseases or syndromes, in order to indicate to people the level of ill health which they are expected to report. Such a check-list always stimulates reporting, sometimes to a degree which is not very useful. In the General Household Survey before 1977, about a quarter to a third of the population declared 'chronic illness', but when in the 1977 edition a check-list was introduced, 56 per cent of men and 70 per cent of women identified themselves as suffering from one or more of the conditions listed.

The most usual way of measuring self-perceived illness, as distinct from the presence or absence of disease, is by means of symptom lists. Commonly, these are related to a relatively brief recall period, and the lists offered may attempt to be exhaustive, covering all possible manifestations of health disturbance (e.g. Hannay 1978), or may simply include a convenient number of the most common symptoms. These subjective indices of health, simple though they may seem, have been shown to have reliable correlations with more objective indicators (Kaplan *et al* 1976,

Hunt and McEwan 1980). They have the advantage of un-covering illness which is not taken for medical diagnosis or treatment, though differential recall, and the possibility that there may be systematic differences in the severity of symptoms that are thought worth reporting, complicate interpretation.

A problem about measuring illness in this way is that its severity, as distinct from its frequency, is not taken into account. One study, a WHO international study of health and health care (Kohn and White 1976), tried to categorize feelings about each symptom the respondents declared. This did not, in fact, sub-stantially alter the patterns of illness found, which, the authors suggested, lent some credibility to the validity of simple symptom lists as a measure. It would seem that, broadly, the number of symptoms suffered in a defined time period is a good indicator of the level of illness experienced by an individual.

Questions on worry or depression are more usually included in instruments specifically designed to measure psycho-social ill health. There are many elaborate, validated instruments for the measurement of psychiatric morbidity (for a review, see Goldberg and Huxley 1980). The concept of psycho-social *health* is less well developed. It shades into a notion of 'social' health, sometimes seen as a third dimension. Referring to the WHO definition of health as 'complete mental, physical and social well-being', for instance, the Alameda County Study (Belloc *et al* 1971) conceptualized health as a spectrum with these three axes, hypothesizing that people would tend to have consistent positions on all three scales.

There is no doubt that health should be defined in the broadest possible terms, and there have been many instruments designed to measure 'quality of life'. It can be argued, how-ever, that this is not quite the same as health. Such measures tend to include the quantity and quality of social resources and social relationships, isolation and integration into the community, life circumstances and life events: there is no doubt that all of these affect health. However, if health itself is defined in this broad social way, then a life change such as bereavement, or social change such as moving to an unfavourable environ-ment, will by definition indicate a change in personal health status. If the purpose of the health indicators – as in the present study – is to provide a tool for the measurement of the effects of

41

social and other circumstances upon health, then this is not very useful.

HEALTH MEASURES USED IN THIS SURVEY

The data available for the measurement of health in the Health and Lifestyle Survey is listed in Appendix A.

From these questions and measurements, four dimensions of health are identified. These are not presented as the only way in which health might be conceptualized. Each is, however, an aspect of health which can be experienced independently from the others, and can (within the information available in the survey) be measured separately. They are:

Unfitness or fitness, based on physiological measurements (called in subsequent tables and diagrams 'unfitness/fitness')

Disease and impairment or their absence, based on reported medically-defined conditions and the degrees of disability which accompany them (called in subsequent tables and diagrams 'disease/disability')

Experienced illness or freedom from illness, based on reports of symptoms suffered (called in subsequent tables and diagrams 'illness')

Psycho-social malaise or well-being, based on reports of psycho-social symptoms (called in subsequent tables and diagrams 'psycho-social health')

For each dimension, as described in Appendix A, individuals were allocated a 'score' on a scale 1–6. Naming the scales presents difficulties, since we have no commonly-accepted words for freedom from illness or the absence of disease. It must be emphasized, however, that they are not simply scales of ill health: each runs from a positive, better than average, state of health, through that which is average, to negative states of ill health. These scales are then used in two ways: separately, to form 'health ratios' by which groups of respondents can be compared, and together, to form 'health categories' by which individuals can be characterized. Before illustrating these, the four dimensions will be considered in turn.

Unfitness/fitness

This is the component which represents health most objectively. It is necessarily limited, since the scale is based on only three measures: blood pressure, lung function, and measured weight for height or body mass index. These three are, however, justified as being measures which have a general significance for health or longevity. Elevated blood pressure is known to be associated with significant extra mortality, principally from cardiovascular and cerebrovascular disease but also from other conditions. Similarly, respiratory function has been shown to be associated with increased mortality from all causes, not only lung diseases. As Ashley *et al* (1975:740) commented, referring to the Framingham Study, ' "vital capacity" literally seems to measure a person's capacity for living'. Finally, those who are overweight are at greater risk of death from all causes, especially coronary heart disease, and also hypertension and diabetes (Royal College of Physicians 1983), and severe underweight may well be an indicator of disease.

Mobility or muscular 'fitness' is not included in this measure. This is in part because the survey has no objective measurement of fitness in this sense, and would have to rely on statements made about abilities and activities. Also, however, functional fitness (being able or unable to work, or to run, or to take part in sports) would appear to be too relative to individual choice or individual circumstances to form part of an objective index. The wheelchair athlete, who considers himself very 'fit', must be borne in mind.

The word 'fitness' is commonly used in several ways, as Chapter 3 noted. Often it has a functional implication – fitness for normal activities – though it frequently has connotations of above-ordinary vigour, physical strength, agility. Among the four health indices being used here, the functional dimension is included in the index of disease and impairment. It must be borne in mind, throughout this analysis, that the dimension which is called 'unfitness/fitness' is defined only as physical fitness, and is restricted to the measures which were available.

Presence/absence of disease and impairment

If 'fitness' is considered as the biological dimension of health, the absence or presence of pathology may be seen as the medical dimension. Since clinical examinations for disease or medical records are not available in this survey, this measure has to rest largely on the answers to the conventional open-ended questions, 'Do you have any long-standing illness, disability or infirmity?' (If yes) 'What is the matter with you?' (Followed by questions about the functional effects of the condition.) Overall, a prevalence of named diseases and impairments of approximately 30 per cent was declared.

The great majority of the more serious conditions (e.g. heart disease, stroke, cancer, liver disease, diabetes, bronchitis, epilepsy and other diseases of the nervous system) were said by the respondents to be 'treated', and thus presumably medically diagnosed. The conditions most likely to be said to be 'untreated', and thus perhaps self-diagnosed, are shown in Table 4.1.

Table 4.1 Conditions (experienced now or in the past) most likely to be 'untreated'

| Condition | Per cent of cases said to be untreated | | | |
	Males (N = 100%)		Females (N = 100%)	
Varicose veins	61	(376)	60	(1,092)
Migraine	49	(541)	38	(1,272)
Haemorrhoids	44	(685)	44	(1,271)
'Back trouble'	32	(1,442)	32	(1,870)
Rheumatism/Arthritis	34	(793)	30	(1,491)

The variety of questions in this survey, combined with the limited information available from the nurses who performed the measurements, enabled some investigation of the reliability of statements about chronic disease to be made. In cases where a particular symptom can be assumed to be closely associated with a particular condition (e.g. 'painful joints' and arthritis/ rheumatism, or 'back pain' and back trouble), those who had said that they suffered currently from the relevant disease were much more likely to complain of the symptom (Table 4.2). On the other hand, less than one third of those people who complained of 'painful joints' and said, when asked specifically, that they had suffered from arthritis, had previously declared arthritis as a chronic condition: in other words, far more people declared a symptom than named a relevant disease. Those who said that they had any chronic condition were more likely than others to be taking prescribed drugs, but a small proportion of people who had not declared any chronic disease were found by the survey nurses to be on long-term medication for such conditions.

Table 4.2 Relationship between declaring a particular symptom, and declaring a relevant disease condition as currently present

Disease	Symptom	Disease declared as present				Disease not declared as present			
		Per cent declaring symptom							
		M	(N)	F	(N)	M	(N)	F	(N)
Arthritis	Painful joints	81	(140)	86	(349)	18	(3,801)	19	(4,749)
'Back trouble'	Back pain	70	(130)	82	(136)	14	(3,811)	19	(4,962)
Bronchitis	Chronic cough	44	(84)	53	(69)	10	(3,821)	10	(5,029)
All mental disorders	'Nerves'/anxiety	49	(51)	74	(85)	6	(3,854)	9	(5,013)

In these cases, the chronic conditions could be added to the individual's record. There is no certainty that every possible case of 'non-reporting' was found in this way, however, and it must be concluded that the accounts obtained about disease in this survey (and, probably, in others) are by no means exhaustive. In particular, it appears that those in non-manual social classes were more ready than those in manual classes to declare that they had a chronic condition, even though it was not function- ally troublesome in any way and was accompanied by no symptoms. Those in manual classes, particularly men, were likely to say that they had a named disease only when it was actually troublesome. Mental disorders were a particular instance of this: few men or women in manual social classes had declared their mental ill health as a chronic condition unless they were currently suffering from 'symptoms'. This may represent a greater reluctance to identify themselves in this way, or may be a diagnostic difference.

In summary, it has to be remembered throughout this analysis that the measure of 'disease' has these limitations. Given that the respondent acknowledged the presence of any chronic condi- tion, however, its 'seriousness', in functional terms, was elicited in what appeared (by internal cross-checks) to be a reliable way by a series of questions about the consequences for the indivi- dual's daily life. The resulting index runs from 'no disease or impairment', through varying degrees of disability, to 'unable to walk and requiring help with the activities of daily living'.

There is, of course, a second dimension to disease: degree of threat. A condition can be serious, in terms of prognosis, without necessarily being currently impairing. The index does not allow for the triviality or life-threatening nature of the condition. It is not always possible, of course, to make valid judgements about severity simply from respondents' descriptions. The importance of this was tested by an examination of an arbitrary selection of named conditions which were likely to be 'serious' or life-threatening, in order to see whether many people with severe but (currently) asymptomatic disease would be likely to be misclassified. In fact, very few with this type of condition claimed that it did not affect their daily lives. There were some with severe impairments, rather than chronic diseases (e.g. blindness), who seemed to be making a deliberate statement by saying that their lives were in no way affected: in these cases it seemed right to accept what they said. In general, however, the severity of conditions appeared to be adequately catered for in the index.

Illness/absence of illness

The basis for the index used to represent this dimension of health is a simple additive score of the number of symptoms experienced 'during the past month'. The list of 16 illness symptoms (see Appendix A: 'symptoms' of psycho-social health such as 'worry' excluded) was selected to represent those which are known to be most common in general populations.

The average number of symptoms, from among the selected 16, which was declared was just over two for men and just under three for women. Six or more different symptoms were claimed by 5 per cent of men and over 10 per cent of women. The prevalence of the most common complaints, at different ages, is shown in Table 4.3, and it can be noted that patterns over the life-course are varied. Many symptoms, such as painful joints or palpitations/breathlessness, rise very steeply with age. Others rise more slowly, or, like headache or colds/flu, actually decline.

Not all possible manifestations of illness are included, of course, for this might be a very long list: the score cannot be held to represent 'the number of symptoms experienced by each

Table 4.3 Prevalence (%) during 'the last month' of some of the most common illness symptoms

	Age 18–24	25–34	35–44	45–54	55–64	65–74	75+
Males							
Painful joints	8	11	16	21	33	28	35
'Bad back'	12	14	17	18	18	17	25
Palpitations/breathlessness	5	4	8	10	20	22	27
Trouble with eyes	10	8	11	13	12	15	25
Trouble with ears	5	4	7	9	12	21	23
Indigestion	12	14	18	18	20	21	18
Headache	25	24	26	19	14	13	13
Cold/flu	40	37	33	27	30	26	27
(N=100%)	(535)	(724)	(745)	(594)	(628)	(448)	(231)
Females							
Painful joints	6	9	16	29	38	43	48
'Bad back'	16	15	19	24	23	28	31
Palpitations/breathlessness	7	8	9	18	22	28	31
Trouble with feet	11	8	12	19	24	23	38
Trouble with ears	6	6	6	9	11	17	22
Indigestion	12	13	15	18	20	23	23
Headache	40	38	38	37	28	25	21
Cold/flu	44	38	29	32	29	27	23
Trouble with periods/ menopause	18	18	23	20	–	–	–
(N=100%)	(625)	(976)	(1,007)	(792)	(762)	(592)	(344)

respondent during a month'. Only diary methods – commonly recording a much higher rate of symptom experience – can do this. The simple score also offers no way, as already discussed, of comparing the severity or chronicity of one person's 'headache' with another's. Nevertheless, the index offers a method of comparing those who appear to suffer frequent illness, and those who experience little or none: considered in relation to self-assessed health status, or to whether or not the individual suffered from declared disease conditions, its face validity was good.

Psycho-social health

The index of psycho-social well-being or malaise, the fourth dimension of health, is similarly based on a simple additive score of symptoms considered to be more psycho-social than physical

– depression, worry, sleep disturbance, feelings of strain, etc. Necessarily, the distinction between symptoms of illness and symptoms of malaise is arbitrary: headache is, for instance, included among the physical illness symptoms, and sleep disturbance among the psycho-social, though neither is invariably so categorized.

The General Health Questionnaire (Goldberg 1972) a screening test for psychiatric disorder, was available for almost three-quarters of the sample. The results produced by the simple score of symptoms were compared with the GHQ, where this was possible, and a good general level of agreement was found. The scale used here is not, however, presented as a psychiatric questionnaire, but only as a measure of self-perceived well-being. High rates of certain individual 'symptoms' were declared, especially among women.

This dimension of health is of course closely associated with personal social circumstances. For the reasons discussed earlier, however, the measure does not include such things as social integration or isolation, contact with family or friends, family or economic circumstances, or personality factors. These are regarded as related to, and perhaps determinants of, psycho-social health, but the measure is independent of them.

Correlation of the four dimensions of health

The simple bivariate correlations of the four health indices are shown in Table 4.4. All four are positively correlated with each other, but often less strongly than might be expected. It is clear that each dimension of health can be experienced separately. Illness and malaise have the strongest association, growing greater with age: it appears that younger people can experience illness without a lack of psycho-social well-being, and vice versa, more easily than the older. Illness and malaise are also highly associated with disease, though here the association rises sharply in middle age rather than showing a smooth relationship with age. A lack of significant correlation between fitness and psycho-social well-being, amongst most age-groups, is perhaps notable, since it seems to contradict much of what the respondents said. In saying 'I am healthy and happy when I am fit', it appears that they meant something more than the restricted definition of physiological fitness represented by the measure used here. Illness and disease are correlated with unfitness, as would be expected, though less clearly among the young: disease at younger ages is less likely to involve degenerative changes.

Table 4.4 Correlation (Spearman's *rho*) of the four different health indices. In each case 3 age-groups shown separately: younger (18–39), mid (40–59), older (60+)

Males		Illness	Psycho-social health	Fitness/ unfitness
Psycho-social health	(Y)	.29**		
	(M)	.33**		
	(O)	.40**		
Fitness/unfitness	(Y)	.02	.00	
	(M)	.07*	.05*	
	(O)	.14**	.14**	
Disease/disability	(Y)	.19**	.14**	.06
	(M)	.28**	.28**	.15*
	(O)	.33**	.29**	.16**
Females				
Psycho-social health	(Y)	.34**		
	(M)	.33**		
	(O)	.44**		
Fitness/unfitness	(Y)	.07*	.02	
	(M)	.12*	.08	
	(O)	.08*	.08*	
Disease/disability	(Y)	.19**	.13**	.10*
	(M)	.33**	.22**	.17**
	(O)	.34**	.25**	.17**

*P<.01; **P<.001

HEALTH RATIOS

Having identified and produced scales for these four dimensions of health, the problem remains of how they are to be used. The method adopted in most of the analyses in the following chapters is to form 'standardized ratios' for each measure. This method is similar to the Standardized Mortality Ratios usually used for the description of differences in death rates, and owes something to the so-called 'ridit' (Relative to an Identified Distribution) method (Kantor and Winkelstein 1969, Belloc *et al* 1971).

The 'standardized health ratio' for any one of the individual components of health represents the relationship of a group to the mean value on each scale found in the population. A value of 100 represents the mean. A lower value (e.g. 80 on the illness scale) represents less ill health than the mean (e.g. this group has 20 per cent less illness than the average), and a higher value (e.g. 115 on the unfitness/fitness scale) represents greater ill health than the mean (e.g. 15 per cent greater unfitness). For each dimension, the lower the figure, the better the relative health.

The major advantage of this method is that the standard or norm of health is not arbitrarily defined, but is derived from the population. Although for some sorts of measure objective standards are laid down – 'normal' blood pressure falls within agreed limits – for others, the normal is more difficult to define. We do not know what a 'normal' rate of illness symptoms is, nor is it easy to provide standards for a 'normal' state of psycho-social well-being. The use of standardized ratios enables 'better than average' health to be identified as easily as ill health.

A further advantage is that the ratios for different dimensions of health can be compared. There is, of course, no logical equivalence of a value on one scale with the same value on another. Transformed into ratios, they are more directly comparable. Also, the ratios can subsequently easily be standardized for age and gender (or any other characteristics) in order to examine the effect of other variables. The health of smokers of a particular age, for instance, can be related to all men or women of that age, or health experience in a particular region of the country can be standardized for the age and gender composition of the region.

Distribution of the dimensions of health

The way in which the ratios change during the life course – that is, not standardized for age or gender – is shown in Figure 4.1. The balance of the four dimensions of health differed between men and women, and obviously varied with age.

At all ages women experienced, or were ready to describe, more illness and a higher level of psycho-social malaise than men. This is, of course, an invariable finding in health surveys. It is commonly suggested that women's socialization and cultural identity make it easier for them to admit to symptoms. It is

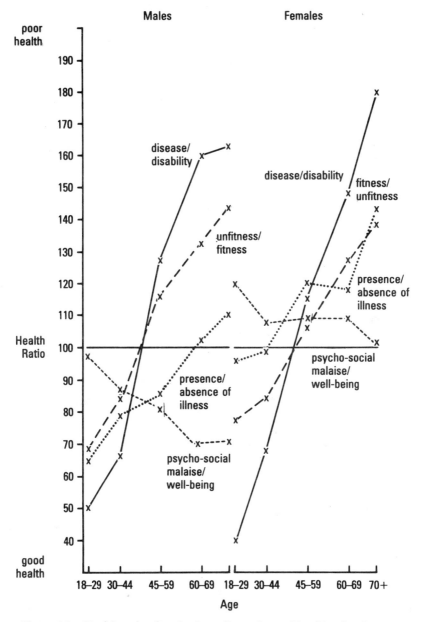

Figure 4.1 Health ratios for the four dimensions of health, showing differences by age and gender (total population mean = 100)

51

certainly possible, however, that physiological differences do mean that women are genuinely more likely to suffer from more minor pain and dysfunction. The contribution of symptoms attributed to menstruation, pregnancy and the menopause (Table 4.3) may be noted. Fitness and the absence or presence of disease, on the other hand, did not differ greatly between the sexes.

Figure 4.1 makes it clear that, as would be expected, it is the relative prevalence of disease and disability which most characterizes ageing. A rise in the experience of illness symptoms was marked for women in middle age, but reversed in the 60s before rising again in old age. One dimension of health – psycho-social well-being – improved with age, if modestly. Again, however, the period between 45 and 59 appears to be one of poorer health for women.

Own assessment of health and health ratios

An example of the use to which these health ratios may be put is shown in Figure 4.2. This demonstrates the relationship between the self-assessments of health as excellent, good, or only fair/poor, which were discussed in Chapter 3, and the four health ratios. Here the ratios are fully standardized for age and gender, and the relative weights of the different components of health can be illustrated. Each dimension is clearly reflected in people's own definition of their health status, though the effect of the presence or absence of disease is the strongest.

All the patterns by age were U-shaped: that is, it was in the middle years that those who defined their health as poor were likely in fact to score poorly, relative to the mean for their age/gender group, on all four measures. Among younger and older men and women there were more likely to be people who assessed their health 'anomalously', so that self-defined excellent and poor health are less clearly separated.

AN OVERALL HEALTH INDEX

The ratio method which has been described is especially useful for comparative purposes. The problem of combining the dimensions of health remains, however: for many purposes, an overall index is required. Who has poor health or all four

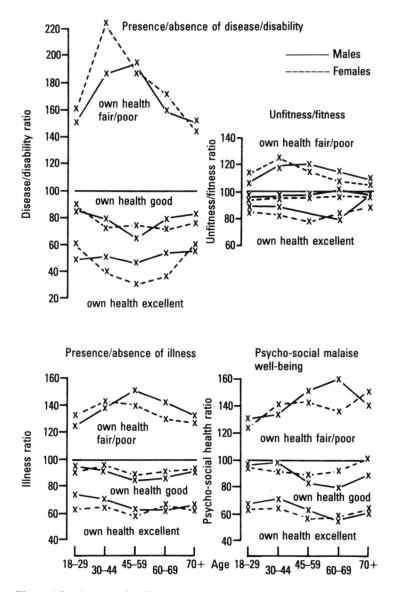

Figure 4.2   Age-standardized health ratios, four dimensions of health, for those who assessed their own health as excellent, good, or fair/poor (all of a given age and gender = 100)

53

dimensions, or health which is above average in every way? Who could be described as unhealthy in one way, but healthy in another?

The simple combination of these ratio scores, or any other form of additive scoring, is rejected: there is no way of demonstrating that a position on one of the scores is equivalent to the same position on others.

The overall health index used here was constructed empirically, by an examination of all the possible combinations of the four health scores. If various degrees of illness/absence of illness, psycho-social malaise/well-being, and unfitness/fitness are considered, together with the presence or absence of disease and its severity or handicapping consequences, there is obviously a very large number of possible health states. In this population, many involved only very few cases. Combining similar categories and those which were rare, eight summary health categories emerged which appear best to represent the data:

1. *Excellent health.* No disease, above average fitness for age (on the limited measures available), and lower than average rates of illness and psycho-social ill health.

2. *Good health.* No disease, at least average fitness, and no more than average illness and psycho-social ill health.

In the following analyses, these two are sometimes combined as 'good' health. It should be noted that good health is defined as accommodating some illness or malaise symptoms, but at a low level. As noted earlier, to experience none at all is highly unusual.

3. *Good health but unfit.* No disease declared and no less than average illness and psycho-social health, but defined as 'unfit', e.g. with poor lung function, and/or measured high blood pressure, and/or underweight or obese.

4. *Good physical health but poor psycho-social health.* No disease, at least average fitness, and low illness, but poorer than average psycho-social health.

5. *High rate of illness without disease.* No disease declared, but a high rate of illness.

6. *'Silent' disease*. Chronic disease declared, but not accompanied by either physical illness or psycho-social ill health.

These four categories represent different kinds of ill health, and cannot be ranked in any order of severity. The final two categories, however, are clearly at the lower end of the health spectrum:

7. *Non-limiting disease and ill*. Chronic disease identified, which is stated to be without functional consequences or disabilities, but with at least average rates of illness and in almost all cases below average fitness.

8. *Limiting disease and ill*. As above, but the chronic disease is accompanied by disabilities or limitations on everyday life.

Distribution of the health categories

'Excellent' and 'good' health, which imply above-average fitness, were associated with youth, as would be expected (Table 4.5). Unlike the 'ratio' method, this way of categorizing people is of course absolute, not relative: in later years individuals may have good health for their age, but it is less likely to be flawless than that of the young and they are less likely to be classified in (1) or (2) above. That 'excellent' health is indeed different from that which is merely 'good' can be tested by noting the proportions of people who were taking prescribed drugs, though the differences are less marked (note especially older women) than might perhaps be expected. These may be compared, however, with the high proportions taking drugs in the 'worst' health category (Table 4.6).

The intermediate health categories are those where there is a shortfall on only one aspect of health. To be unfit, though otherwise in good health, is of course more common as one ages: even if without disease or illness, the old are more likely to be unfit. On the other hand, the group with poor psycho-social health only were more likely to be younger, and women were more likely to come into this category than men. A high rate of illness without disease, and its converse, disease without any symptoms, were not strongly age-related, though since women (as shown previously) tend to perceive or declare more illness symptoms, they were more likely, especially when young, to come into the 'illness only' category.

55

Table 4.5 Distribution of combined health categories by age and gender (per cent)

Health category	Males				
	Age 18–29	30–44	45–59	60–69	70+
Excellent	19	11	5	4	2
Good	34	33	23	18	16
Good but unfit	7	11	17	16	18
Good but poor psycho-social health	14	10	7	3	3
High illness without disease	7	9	7	7	8
'Silent' disease	7	9	15	15	12
Poor, non-limiting disease	5	8	10	13	16
Very poor, limiting disease	6	7	17	23	24
(N = 100%)	(738)	(986)	(772)	(452)	(361)

Health category	Females				
	Age 18–29	30–44	45–59	60–69	70+
Excellent	10	9	5	3	3
Good	31	31	20	15	10
Good but unfit	6	8	10	14	13
Good but poor psycho-social health	21	14	10	8	4
High illness without disease	17	13	14	12	12
'Silent' disease	4	6	6	9	8
Poor, non-limiting disease	6	9	14	17	18
Very poor, limiting disease	5	9	18	23	32
(N = 100%)	(879)	(1,318)	(926)	(562)	(414)

Table 4.6 Proportions taking prescribed drugs in different health categories (per cent)

Health category	Males			Females		
	Age 18–39	40–59	60+	18–39	40–59	60+
Excellent	2	7	19	9	9	29
Good	5	12	26	14	18	23
Very poor	42	73	87	58	74	88

When the physiological fitness of younger people in the 'illness without disease' group was examined, poor lung function emerged as the best marker, among the measures available, of a high rate of illness for which no disease label had been offered. Among men and women over 60, high measured blood pressure similarly distinguished this group.

The specific conditions involved in the category of 'silent' disease – disease which is said to be without any functional consequences and is without a high rate of illness symptoms – included many with an obvious status of disease or impairment without illness: 40 per cent of those with skin diseases came into this category, 31 per cent of those with sight problems, 29 per cent of those with hearing problems, and 23 per cent of those with orthopaedic impairments that did not affect mobility.

Finally, the two categories of undoubtedly poor health rise steeply with age, as would be expected.

Own assessment of health and health categories

An example of the use of these categories is, again, to relate them to self-assessments (Table 4.7). There is a clear trend towards 'appropriate' assessments at the extremes: those in the best categories of 'measured' health were not likely to say that their health was poor, and those in the worst were less likely to say that it was good. However, it has to be noted that 10 per cent of men and 7 per cent of women in the best health category still said that their health was only poor or fair, and at the other extreme as many as 40 per cent of those with undoubtedly poor health claimed that it was good. The evidence of the health ratio analysis (Figure 4.2) is supplemented by the demonstration that, among the 'good' categories of health, the elderly are more likely to judge their health favourably than the young: the norm of what it is to experience excellent health is obviously less stringent as age increases. At the other extreme, to have a chronic disease is more likely to be seen as poor health if the condition is accompanied by functional limitations, as might be expected, but the experience of illness symptoms is also extremely salient.

Some of the intermediate categories offer further evidence about what the respondents saw as good or bad health. For instance, low psycho-social well-being, even among those without physical symptoms or disease conditions, was readily defined as poor health. It is perhaps of interest that this is particularly true among men: women are more likely to appear in this

Table 4.7 Proportion of those within different combined categories of health who assess their own health as only fair/poor (per cent of age group)

Health category	Males				Females			
	Age 18–39	40–59	60+	*(N all ages)*	*Age* 18–39	40–59	60+	*(N all ages)*
Excellent	13	5	1	(314)	8	5	1	(283)
Good	20	13	13	(891)	16	7	11	(994)
Poor	31	35	33	(311)	28	38	34	(474)
Very poor	47	65	60	(562)	61	63	62	(685)
	All ages							
Good but unfit		17		(391)		15		(388)
Good but poor psycho-social health		34		(290)		27		(535)
High illness without disease		33		(264)		35		(577)
'Silent' disease		27		(244)		23		(163)

Table 4.8 Assessment of own health related to 'measured' combined health categories in non-manual and manual social classes (per cent of social class group who assess their own health as only fair/poor)

Health category	Males		Females	
	Non-man.	*Man.*	*Non-man.*	*Man.*
Excellent/good	10	17	10	12
Poor/very poor	39	56*	43	57*
Good but unfit	12	17	10	19*
Good but poor psycho-social health	27	39*	23	30
Illness without disease	31	38	25	38*
'Silent' disease	21	24	21	24

Difference between non-manual and manual by χ^2: *$P<.01$

category, but less likely, when they do, to call their health poor. 'Silent' disease, on the other hand, was less readily identified as poor health among both men and women.

If the two broad social classes – non-manual families and manual, classified by the occupation of the husband in the case of married couples – are distinguished, Table 4.8 shows that those people in manual families were, in general, rather more likely to take a 'pessimistic' view of their health. If their health was, on all the available evidence, good, they were more likely to call it poor, and if they were in fact unhealthy they were less likely to claim, optimistically, that it was good. It is of course probable, and is a topic to be investigated in the next chapter, that health is generally class-related. What are the correlates of poor health in less-advantaged circumstances, however, which are likely to make poor health 'feel' subjectively worse or encourage a pessimistic view? Chapter 5 may offer some clues.

Chapter Five

SOCIAL CIRCUMSTANCES AND HEALTH

Using the measures described in Chapter 4, the association of health with people's social circumstances will be considered.

Of course, health has long served as a barometer of the economic and social conditions under which people live. This is clearest where conditions are worst: poor housing, especially damp housing, lack of adequate heating or other facilities, a poorer environment in terms of pollution of accident risks, hazardous or punishing work, the bad diet of poverty, these can all be readily seen as likely to affect health. There is considerable evidence that material deprivation affects the development of young children, and that the effects of this can continue into adult life.

More general relationships between health and economic and social circumstances, not confined to those in extreme poverty, have usually been demonstrated in terms of premature death. As noted in Chapter 1, mortality is easier to measure than health. But the evidence of mortality suggests that the issue is not simply one of the disadvantage associated with extreme deprivation, but of a general and structured association between prosperity and privilege and health experience.

It must be made clear that the evidence of this chapter can in no way be taken to prove cause and effect. It may well be that poverty, or worse environments, or particular types of occupation, or unemployment, or social isolation, are directly detrimental to health. It may also be, however, that those whose health is poorest are most likely to be downwardly mobile in occupational terms, or to become unemployed, or to be least successful both economically and socially. Issues such as these are discussed in the final chapter. Here, all that is being shown is the nature and the magnitude of any associations between social circumstances and health.

Social class

Social class, viewed as a distributional measure, is the most commonly used index of social circumstances. A great deal is known about the relationship between mortality and class, especially through the Registrar General's Decennial Reports. Of recent years there has been much discussion about whether class differences in rates of premature death may not actually be increasing. Less firm information has been available about morbidity, or class patterns of general health status, though the General Household Survey has always shown a steep gradient through the social classes for declared 'limiting long-standing illness', with the rates in the unskilled manual group more than double those in the professional group for both men and women.

Social class, as defined by the Registrar General in terms of occupation, is of course a summary measure. It implies differences in income, education, environment, power over resources, and behaviour, but measures none of them directly: it can perhaps best be regarded simply as a starting point for the investigation of social circumstances and health.

The major classification used here is the conventional Registrar General social class, based on occupation, or previous occupation in the case of the retired, or husband's occupation in the case of married women. This leaves a small proportion – those who have never had an occupation – unclassified, and presents well-known problems in the case of married women. In the Health and Lifestyle Survey, the relationship between a classification for married women based on their husband's occupation, and a classification based on their own occupation or previous occupation, was examined in detail. For most 'lifestyle' characteristics – levels of family income, housing, and even some behavioural characteristics such as diet or social activities – the use of husband's occupation produced clearer trends. The conventional measure of social class also produced stronger relationships with health. The explanation lies in the large proportion of married women, especially those in part-time employment, working in jobs 'below' their educational standard, when compared to their husbands. At a broad level, the important distinction appeared to be whether married women were working outside the home or not, rather than the nature of their jobs. (This raises questions, of course about the meaning of employment and unemployment for married women, which will be discussed later.) Because the husband's occupation appeared better to represent the social characteristics of the couple, however, and because of the large number of married women who could not be classified by a current job, the conventional Registrar General's social class method is the one principally used here. This does not imply that women's own jobs are irrelevant to their health, however, and these will sometimes be used as an alternative classification.

Considering the overall health categories of Table 4.5, the likelihood of good or poor health was strongly class-related in the Health and Lifestyle population, after the age of 40. This is demonstrated in Table 5.1, where classes I/II (professional, employers and managerial families), class III non-manual (other non-manual occupations), class III manual (skilled manual occupations and own-account tradesmen), and classes IV/V (service occupations, semi-skilled and unskilled) are distinguished. (Classes I/II and classes IV/V are combined because of relatively small numbers, in some age-groups, in class I and class V.) Differences were particularly marked in middle age. Expressed as an odds ratio, men of 40–59 in social classes I/II were 1.73 times as likely to be in good overall health as men in classes IV/V. For the likelihood of poor health there was little social differentiation among women, however, and among men the major distinction, in the middle and older ages, was between those in professional and managerial classes, and all the rest.

The class distribution of some of the intermediate or 'anomalous' health categories (p. 54) is of interest. Low psycho-social well-being without physical symptoms shows a difference between classes only for younger women, with 23 per cent of class IV/V women aged 18–39 in this category, but only 14 per cent of class I/II women. Otherwise the experience of this type of ill health appears to be a personal phenomenon, unrelated to class. A high rate of illness symptoms without any declared disease, on

Table 5.1 Social class distribution of health categories, per cent of age/
social class group

Health category	Age	Males Social class I/II	IIIN	IIIM	IV/V	Females I/II	IIIN	IIIM	IV/V
Good/excellent	18–39	48	53	48	48	46	41	41	35
	40–59	39	37	28	27	35	33	30	22
	60+	24	19	20	18	20	18	14	10
Poor/very poor	18–39	12	15	13	12	15	14	15	13
	40–59	17	25	29	29	28	27	31	30
	60+	33	38	39	40	41	44	46	45
Good but unfit	All	8	10	12	12	10	11	13	15
Good but poor psycho-social health	All	9	7	8	7	10	13	11	14
High illness without disease	All	7	7	9	11	11	13	14	18
'Silent' disease	All	16	13	9	10	8	8	6	5
(N = 100%)	(18–39)	(364)	(198)	(517)	(292)	(491)	(324)	(585)	(384)
	(40–59)	(329)	(115)	(406)	(220)	(474)	(143)	(428)	(256)
	(60+)	(215)	(84)	(304)	(207)	(242)	(128)	(341)	(245)

the other hand, shows marked class trends at all ages and for
both men and women, with manual classes more likely than non-
manual to have described this sort of ill health. The only health
category which shows a reverse class gradient is that which was
called 'silent' disease, or chronic conditions without symptoms or
functional consequences. Given the nature of the conditions described, as noted in Chapter 4, it seems likely that this demonstrates a greater readiness on the part of non-manual respondents
to name a chronic condition, even if it is not troublesome in any
way, rather than a lower prevalence of disease.

A more detailed examination of each component of health
separately, using the Relative Health Index method, is illustrated in Figure 5.1. Here narrower age-groups are used, and
indices are completely age and gender standardized. Thus the
comparison is only between social classes: an index of over 100
means not that a particular group had a worse-than-average
experience of ill health than the overall mean, but that health on
that dimension was relatively poorer compared only with all of
the same age in other social classes.

It can be noted that at all ages, and for each dimension of
health, there was a tendency for experience to be poorer as

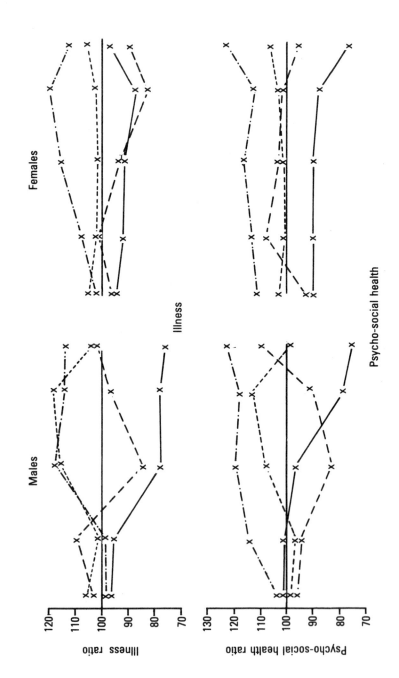

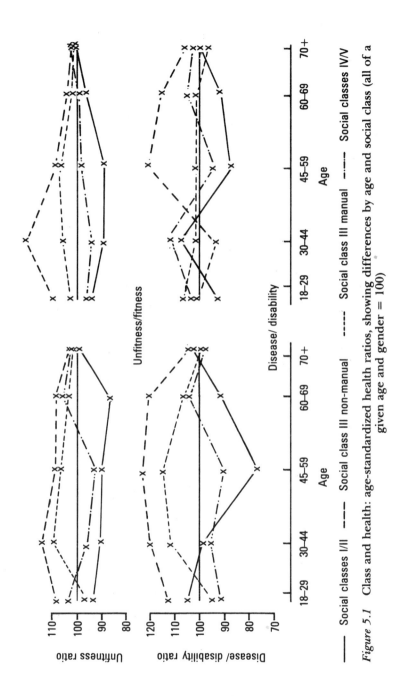

Figure 5.1 Class and health: age-standardized health ratios, showing differences by age and social class (all of a given age and gender = 100)

social class declined. At the start of adult life, differences between social classes did exist, but they were small and not always quite regular – for instance, among young men the professional/employers/managerial group, social classes I/II, did not have the best psycho-social health nor the lowest rate of disease. The effect of social circumstances, as life progresses (and ill health becomes more common), is clear. By the middle years, differences for all the dimensions of health were wide and regular. For men, but not for women, there was a tendency for gaps to develop particularly between the non-manual groups, classes I/II and III non-manual, and the manual groups, the skilled workers of class III manual and the semi- and unskilled of classes IV/V. It can also be noted that the dimension of fitness showed divergence between classes, for both men and women, at a rather earlier age than the other components of health. Over 60, and especially over 70, class differences in the more subjective dimensions of health – illness and psycho-social health – continued to be great, and indeed it was amongst the most elderly people that psycho-social health differed most. For the more objective dimensions – fitness and disease – the classes converged, so that in old age there was even less difference than there had been in youth. At the oldest ages, there is of course some possibility of a healthy survivor effect, with those who might have been least fit in their middle years – disproportionately among manual social classes – less likely to survive.

Occupation

Since social class, defined in this broad way, is a proxy for the effects of so many socio-economic and other differences, it is possible that the true extent of health differences is concealed. Each class is made up of widely different occupations (as can be demonstrated, in health terms, by mortality rates), and this heterogeneity may mean that the real impact of socio-economic differences is smoothed out. Studies of single occupations have found steeper gradients in mortality than are shown in national social class data. For instance, in the Whitehall study of civil servants (Marmot *et al* 1984), there was a greater than three-fold difference in mortality rates between the highest and lowest grades, a much greater difference within one type of occupation than exists, overall, between the highest and the lowest of the Registrar General's social classes.

Occupations are therefore more finely distinguished in Table 5.2, where only those currently working are included, and both men and women are categorized by their own occupation. The occupational groupings known as 'socio-economic groups' are used rather than actual occupations, since numbers otherwise become small. Thus the overall range demonstrated is not necessarily greater than it was for the social classes. However, differences concealed within broad social class classifications can be noted: for instance, among younger men (but not older) the considerable difference between employers/managers in large establishments and those in small. The health of skilled, or even semi-skilled, manual workers was, by the multi-dimensional measure used here, more likely to be generally good than that of 'small' employers. Younger personal service workers, though shown as likely to have 'good' health, were also more likely than others to be categorized as 'poor psycho-social health, though good physical health' (21 per cent of this occupation, compared with 13 per cent of all men aged 18–39). Foremen/supervisors, and own-account tradesmen, show relatively poor health at all ages, and both were prominent in the 'poor psycho-social health' and 'high illness without disease' categories. The good health of young agricultural workers can be noted, though it was not sustained in the older group. (It must be borne in mind, however, that some of the special occupational groups mentioned above are represented by relatively low numbers.)

Among younger employed women, there are certain types of occupation – professional and intermediate non-manual, own-account trades – where the health 'profiles' seem very similar to those of men in the same occupations. Among employers/ managers they were 'better', but in other occupations – junior non-manual, personal service, manual workers whether skilled or not – they were conspicuously 'worse'. It is among these latter occupations that women's greater likelihood of being categorized as 'frequent illness without disease' takes them out of the overall 'very healthy' category. Over 40, in contrast to men, women's health did not appear to be strongly associated with their own occupations.

It seems likely that these associations, for women, are not

Table 5.2 Proportions in 'good' and 'poor' health categories, working men and women according to occupation (per cent)

Occupation	Males			Females		
	Health category					
	Good/ Ex.	Poor/V. poor	(N = 100%)	Good/ Ex.	Poor/V. poor	(N = 100%)
Age 18–39						
Employer/manager (large)	51	11	(98)	54	9	(55)
Employer/manager (small)	38	19	(112)	49	14	(100)
Professional	47	10	(70)	47	11	(57)
Intermediate non-manual	49	12	(130)	48	13	(144)
Junior non-manual	58	15	(150)	43	14	(232)
Personal service	58	12	(33)	44	17	(47)
Foreman/supervisor	41	12	(51)	42	19	(37)
Skilled manual	50	12	(362)	40	15	(206)
Semi-skilled manual	47	12	(170)	35	19	(122)
Unskilled manual	39	16	(62)	35	19	(33)
Own-account trades	45	15	(75)	42	19	(62)
Agricultural	61	9	(34)	+	+	
Age 40–59						
Employer/manager (large)	44	18	(90)	37	23	(80)
Employer/manager (small)	41	14	(111)	36	23	(107)
Professional	34	12	(59)	32	32	(57)
Intermediate non-manual	38	17	(95)	36	24	(86)
Junior non-manual	39	18	(75)	31	20	(86)
Personal service	+	+		+	+	
Foreman/supervisor	34	25	(64)	26	21	(43)
Skilled manual	31	24	(227)	31	23	(167)
Semi-skilled manual	33	20	(116)	27	24	(96)
Unskilled manual	30	a2	(51)	30	26	(34)
Own-account trades	35	20	(49)	35	22	(49)
Agricultural	39	27	(33)	+	+	

+ base number <30

entirely causal relationships. In some cases they may be: for instance, it is possible that some occupations classified as 'skilled manual' are less conducive to health for women than for men. For the most part, however, it is probable that what is being demonstrated is selection into and out of the labour market. In younger years, those women with non-manual jobs are likely to be the healthier. In later years, the less healthy leave the labour market (an exception may be women in professional occupations, shown in Table 5.2 to include many in poor health after 40), so that there is more uniformity among those who are still working outside the home than there is among men.

When compared with men in the same type of occupation, women in manual classes often appear in Table 5.2 to have as great a likelihood of good health as men, although when the same comparison is made by social class they are less likely. It seems probable that this is not only due to selection out of work of the less healthy, but also related to the fact that many married women work, especially part-time, at jobs which are 'downgraded'. The health of women working in unskilled jobs in the Health and Lifestyle Survey, for instance, was no worse than that of those in semi-skilled work: this was not true of men. The same phenomenon has been observed in relation to mortality rates (Fox and Goldblatt 1982).

Income

Income, closely associated with occupation, is obviously an important dimension of the social class structure. Again, however, as Wilkinson (1986b) has shown, 'If we take income as a reasonable indicator of people's standards of living, it is clear that there are neither the differences between classes nor the homogeneity within classes that we might expect to find'. Income data show that, while classes I and II tend to be clearly separated from the others, class IIIM has the next highest median incomes and there are only trivial differences between the other classes (OPCS 1986).

Thus the questions may be asked: are differences in health experience greater by income than by social class? And to what extent do the social class differences represent simply material standards of living, determined by poverty or prosperity, and to what extent are other dimensions of class involved?

It must be borne in mind that the measure of household income used here is necessarily crude. It was not practicable to enquire about all sources of income in detail, and the estimates which were declared have not been adjusted for size of household. Those people who did not know the total income of the household they were living in (principally young people living with their parents or others, but including also some married women) are excluded; there was also some refusal to answer this question.

However, Figure 5.2 gives a simple demonstration of the

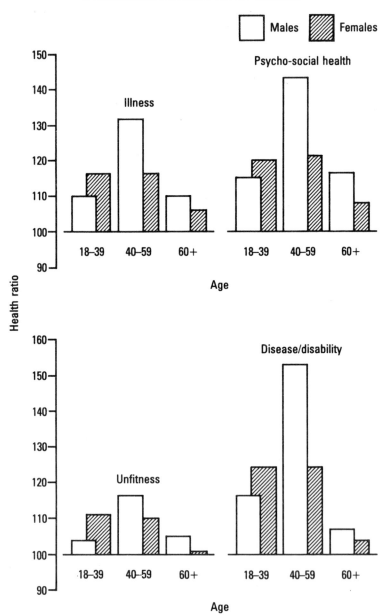

Figure 5.2 Income and health: age-standardized health ratios for those with a low household income (£100/week or less) (all of a given age and gender, all incomes, = 100)

importance of income. About a quarter of those who did declare a household income named a figure of £100/week or less: these are arbitrarily selected out as 'low-income' respondents. A high proportion were over 60 years of age, as might be expected. Figure 5.2 shows the health ratios, standardized for gender and for age within broad life-stages, for this group. It can be noted that there are remarkably regular patterns. Young women of this low-income group tended to have relatively poorer health then men, in all four dimensions of health. Over 40, however, the health of low-income men was more likely to be relatively poor than that of women, and particularly disadvantaged in the middle years of 40–59. For this age-group of men, the health deficit associated with low income appears to be greater than that associated with social class. At all ages and for both men and women, however, the health of those in low-income households was clearly poorer than the population average.

In order to provide a statistical estimate of the importance of income, in relation to other aspects of social class, a series of multivariate analyses was performed. From these, odds can be derived which indicate the likelihood of low income being associated with poor health if class is taken into account, or the effect of class isolated from income. Table 5.3 shows the odds on having higher than average illness, or poorer than average psycho-social health, considering arbitrarily-defined 'low' and 'high' incomes (with a dividing line of £580/month) and the two broadly distinguished social classes, manual and non-manual. For most age-gender groups, income carried more weight than social class. The only group in which social class modestly but significantly raised the likelihood of greater illness, when income group was taken into account, was young women. For both men and women in the middle and older years, the odds on high illness for the lower income group, with social class taken into account, were 1.3 or 1.4 to one. The effect of the interaction of income and social class among men, though not great enough to reach significance, was always negative: that is, to have a low income and manual social class was not quite as disadvantageous as the individual effects might suggest. For women in the middle years, this negative interaction was strong enough to have a statistically significant effect.

For psycho-social health, low income, independently of social

71

Table 5.3 Odds ratios (loglinear analysis): association of social class and income with illness and psycho-social health

	Males			Females		
	Age 18–39	40–59	60+	18–39	40–59	60+
Odds on high level of illness						
Social class – manual:non-manual	NS	NS	NS	1.18	NS	NS
Income – low:high	NS	1.37	1.39	1.19	1.35	1.33
Interaction of social class and income	NS	NS	NS	NS	.83	NS
Odds on low level of psycho-social health						
Social class – manual:non-manual	NS	NS	1.38	NS	1.23	NS
Income – low:high	1.15	1.40	1.32	1.38	1.37	1.34
Interaction of social class and income	NS	NS	NS	NS	NS	NS

class, increased the likelihood of greater malaise for both men and women of all ages. For this dimension of health, low social class of itself increased malaise significantly only for older men and, to a lesser extent, women in the middle years. Thus these analyses support the conclusion that the apparently strong association of social class and health is primarily an association of income and health.

The shape of this relationship is unlikely to be a straight line. Successive increases in income are likely to bring diminishing returns, in health or any other advantage: to double an income of £100/week may be presumed to make more difference than adding £100 to an income many times this size. Wilkinson (1986b) has demonstrated this curvilinear relationship between income and mortality rates. In Figure 5.3, the 'effect' of successive increments of £50/week is illustrated, selecting as examples the age-group 40–59 and the three dimensions of health which Figure 5.2 showed were most clearly associated with income. It is obvious that the 'return' on equal increments does indeed diminish: in most cases, there is no improvement in the health ratios after the fourth or fifth point on the scale. Indeed, the fifth point (representing average incomes of approximately £250/week) tends to be the 'healthiest'. A perhaps surprising result of this analysis was the small, but quite regular, rise in ill

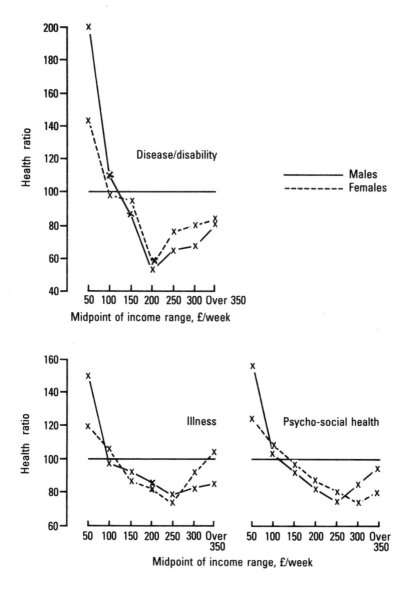

Figure 5.3 Income and health: age-standardized health ratios, illness and psycho-social health, in relation to weekly income, demonstrating the effect of £50/week increments in household income, males and females age 40–59 (all of a given age and gender = 100)

health of all kinds at the high-income end of the scale. Is it true that a moderately high income is more conducive to health than a very high one? This is a point to be considered when examining patterns of behaviour later in this analysis. What is certain, however, is that low incomes are strongly associated with poorer health.

Region

The well-publicized NW/SE 'divide' in health in Britain rests largely, like the social class divide, on mortality figures. The regional trends are in part a reflection of the different social class compositions of regions, but remain even when social class is taken into account. The social class gap is greatest where overall death rates are highest, e.g. the mortality rate of men aged 20–64 in social class IV/V is 188 per cent of that of men in social class I/II in the northern region, and 143 per cent in East Anglia. Nevertheless, within social classes the geographical divide remains.

The age-composition of regions also varies, which will affect typical health experience as well as crude mortality rates. In Figure 5.4, England, Wales and Scotland are divided into three broad regions, and the relative health ratios in the Health and Lifestyle sample, completely standardized for age, are shown for non-manual and manual classes compared for each of the health dimensions. (Greater London has been excluded from the surrounding South East because in many ways it appears to demonstrate different health patterns.)

This method of demonstrating the way in which different components of health differ offers some interesting results. In general, health was better in the South and East, for all dimensions, than in the North or the West and Midlands. The West and Midlands produced the poorest ratios for illness in men, and for unfitness in both men and women, but otherwise it was in the North that the average level of health was worst. Differences between broad regions were least for the prevalence of disease, and not very great for illness among women: these are results that the ratio method might be expected to emphasize, since disease rates are high among the elderly, wherever they live, and illness rates higher among all women than men. The regional differences demonstrated are not, however, due to different age-compositions of the areas, since the ratios are age-standardized, nor are they due to the weight of manual occupations in the North. Non-manual and manual families are distinguished, and in each region the health of manual men and women was poorer for every dimension. (It must be noted, however, that this simple distinction may not allow for the differential distribution of levels of occupation *within* the broad social classes.)

The result of the combined effect of region and social class is that, in general, the typical level of health of a man in manual social classes in the South and East was equal to, or in the case of fitness better than, that of a non-manual man in the North. The extent of social class differences was not, however, the same throughout the country. For men (with the exception of the illness dimension) class differences were smallest in the South and East, and tended to be greatest in the West and Midlands. For women, on the other hand, class differences in the more subjective measures of illness and psycho-social health were greatest in the South and East.

Small areas

'Region', like social class, is obviously a variable with many dimensions, involving not only different occupations and age-structures, but also incomes, levels of unemployment, housing, and qualities of the physical environment, as well as those characteristics which are more clearly 'geographical', such as climate. As with social class, there is evidence that there is greater heterogeneity within Standard Regions than there is between them. Research has suggested that it is material deprivation *within* regions that is associated with health. For instance, Townsend *et al.* (1985, 1986) demonstrated that the healthiest areas in the Northern Region compared well with the healthiest areas in Bristol. In the Northern Region a composite health index was used, including rates of permanent sickness and disability as well as mortality and the birth of low birthweight babies. The correspondence of this health index with an index of deprivation (income, housing, unemployment, etc.) was extremely close at the level of districts, and the variation not

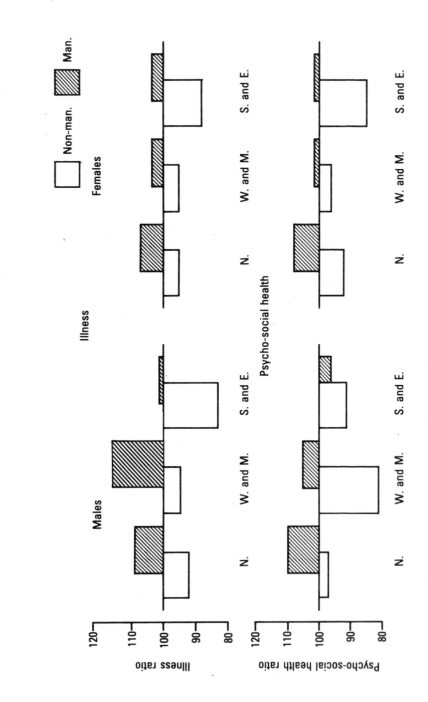

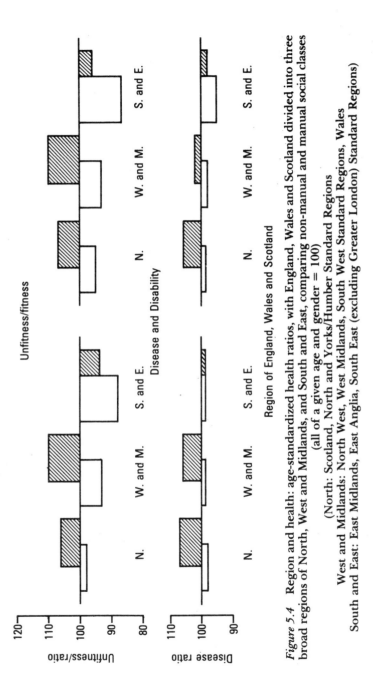

Figure 5.4 Region and health: age-standardized health ratios, with England, Wales and Scotland divided into three broad regions of North, West and Midlands, and South and East, comparing non-manual and manual social classes (all of a given age and gender = 100)

(North: Scotland, North and Yorks/Humber Standard Regions
West and Midlands: North West, West Midlands, South West Standard Regions, Wales
South and East: East Midlands, East Anglia, South East (excluding Greater London) Standard Regions)

altogether 'explained' by social class. Similar findings relating to small areas, have been shown in, for instance, Glasgow and Edinburgh (Carstairs 1981, Boddy and Forbes 1981), Sheffield (Thunhurst 1985) and London (Townsend *et al.* 1986).

A useful tool for the investigation of small area, rather than regional, differences is the socio-economic classification of local authority areas of Craig (1985). Forty variables – demographic and household structure, housing, socio-economic structure, and employment – are used empirically to uncover 30 'clusters' which describe any area in England, Wales and Scotland. These are then combined to form six 'families'. Four of the families can be divided into two, giving a ten-family classification. For the most part, a six-family schema, described in Table 5.4, is used for the Health and Lifestyle data, since otherwise numbers may become small. 'Mixed areas with industry' and 'traditional manufacturing areas' are combined, as are Inner and Central London, and 'rural' and 'resort and retirement' areas.

Table 5.4 Health ratios in 'small areas', standardized for the age and sex composition of areas

| | Area | | | | | |
	1	2	3	4	5	6
	Males					
Illness	96	93	108	105	92	100
Psycho-social health	96	84	108	105	110	120
Fitness	94	104	102	107	98	97
Disease/disability	87	100	109	109	99	98
(N)	(789)	(686)	(907)	(479)	(272)	(174)
	Females					
Illness	96	91	105	119	95	112
Psycho-social health	95	91	106	104	100	119
Fitness	94	99	101	106	102	102
Disease/disability	89	96	107	111	87	107
(N)	(939)	(863)	(1149)	(603)	(330)	(215)

Small areas
1 Established high status areas, higher status growth areas ('high status')
2 More rural areas, resort and retirement areas ('rural/resort')
3 Mixed, areas with some industry, traditional manufacturing areas ('industrial')
4 Service centres and cities ('cities')
5 Areas with much local authority housing, new towns ('L.A. areas')
6 Inner and Central London ('London')

The differences between the 'families' of small areas are shown to be similar in magnitude to those between the broad regions. The families show more clearly, however, the sort of social and environmental factors which appear to be most important. The health of people living in high-status areas (family 1) was better than average, for every dimension, wherever in the country they were situated. In rural and resort areas the dimensions of illness and psycho-social health were even more favourable, though not, for men, the dimensions of disease and unfitness (the age-structure of these areas tends of course to be high, but this is taken into account by the age standardization of the ratios). Health was generally at its worst in industrial areas (family 3), and in cities and service centres (family 4), with notably high levels of illness for women in cities. London (family 6) differed from the other city areas for men in that disease and unfitness were less, but psycho-social health was particularly poor. For women in London, all the dimensions of health – and again, particularly psycho-social health – were unfavourable. New towns and other areas with a high proportion of local authority housing (family 5) had lower than average rates of illness, and of disease for women, but also appeared to be characterized by poor psycho-social health for men.

Of course, these overall figures may conceal many finer differences. Different types of area are more, or less, common in different geographical regions; they contain different mixes of occupational classes; the 'effect' of the living environment may not be the same for the young and the old. Is it 'better', from a health point of view, to belong to the more advantaged social classes and live in industrial areas, or to be a manual worker and live in a 'healthier' environment? Is the poor health of industrial areas concentrated among the young, or is it due to people becoming unhealthy in their later years? Are rural areas equally healthy in the North and the South? The answers to these questions may go some way to distinguishing between the importance of those elements of lifestyle which are typical of socio-economic status, and those elements which are truly regional or associated with the external living environment.

An attempt was made to consider these questions by breaking down each area by broad non-manual or manual social class, representing the socio-economic dimension, and by age-groups.

There are, of course, many other variables which might be relevant. For instance, income within social classes is not considered, and it is possible that this may vary by area. The manual worker living in a 'high status' area may, typically, have a different type of occupation to the worker who lives in one of the traditional industrial areas. Thus the conclusions presented

Table 5.5 Health ratios for selected small areas and age groups, by social class (standardized for age within groups)

	Males				Females			
	Non-man.	Man.	(N)		Non-man.	Man.	(N)	
Illness, age 18–39								
High status	98	108	(175)	(165)	84	112	(243)	(191)
Rural/resort	98	98	(104)	(131)	99	98	(142)	(178)
Industrial	102	105	(142)	(277)	98	105	(186)	(334)
Illness, age 40–59								
High status	90	97	(131)	(133)	92	96	(172)	(134)
Rural/resort	78	84	(101)	(116)	81	107	(164)	(134)
Cities	109	121	(58)	(117)	124	115	(68)	(117)
Psycho-social health, age 18–39								
High status	98	102	(175)	(165)	90	118	(243)	(191)
Industrial	108	113	(142)	(277)	107	112	(186)	(334)
London	136	107	(46)	(36)	118	103	(65)	(40)
Psycho-social health, age 40–59								
Rural/resort	79	78	(101)	(116)	98	102	(164)	(134)
Industrial	91	119	(89)	(180)	99	134	(151)	(215)
Cities	112	105	(58)	(117)	136	144	(68)	(117)
Fitness, age 18–39								
Rural/resort	103	101	(104)	(131)	98	103	(142)	(178)
Industrial	97	108	(142)	(277)	100	102	(186)	(334)
L.A. areas	70	123	(48)	(76)	85	113	(66)	(82)
Fitness, age 40–59								
High status	81	100	(131)	(133)	86	95	(172)	(134)
Industrial	96	112	(89)	(180)	87	120	(151)	(215)
Cities	101	112	(58)	(117)	94	113	(68)	(117)
Disease/disability, age 18–59								
High status	79	83	(306)	(398)	78	91	(415)	(325)
Industrial	118	113	(231)	(457)	122	101	(337)	(549)
Cities	109	115	(130)	(231)	106	113	(180)	(261)
Disease/disability, age 60+								
Rural/resort	74	91	(99)	(119)	80	96	(132)	(96)
Industrial	102	115	(62)	(147)	94	132	(73)	(172)
Cities	93	119	(29)	(84)	120	112	(43)	(112)

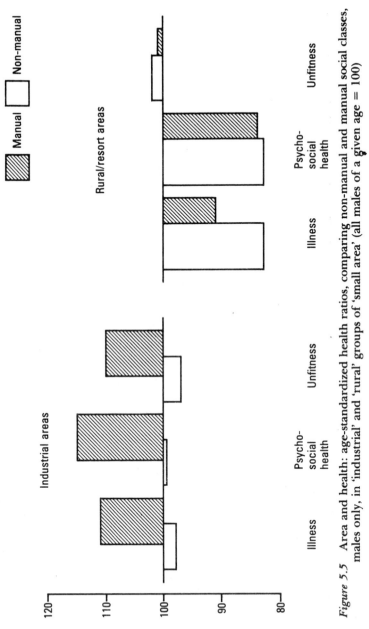

Figure 5.5 Area and health: age-standardized health ratios, comparing non-manual and manual social classes, males only, in 'industrial' and 'rural' groups of 'small area' (all males of a given age = 100)

in Table 5.5 and Figure 5.5 can be no more than suggestive: they do, however, suggest some previously unexamined and interesting relationships.

Table 5.5 presents health ratios for the two broad social classes, in different age-groups, comparing selected area 'families'. Although, as already established, the health of manual men and women was almost always poorer than that of non-manual, it is clear that types of living area do make a considerable difference. In cities, illness among women in manual classes, in the middle years, was in fact less than that experienced by non-manual women, for instance. Disease and disability was considerably less among manual families living in high status areas than among non-manual men and women in industrial areas.

However, the difference between classes varied in the different areas. For men in 'high status', i.e. 'good' residential areas, non-manual men had better ratios than manual. For women, class differences were also relatively wide, especially for the dimensions of illness and psycho-social health. Psycho-social health, for young manual women, was poorer in high status areas than in any other type of area. Explanations for this can only be speculative: perhaps they lie in the area of social support and family structures, less cohesive in 'suburban' than in 'traditional' areas. Certainly, it is not due to higher proportions of those women whose situations, as will be shown, appear to make them particularly vulnerable to psycho-social malaise – such as single-handed parents – since these groups, like the very poor, are under-represented in the areas described as 'high status'.

In industrial areas, similarly, class differences were wide for both men and women. Rates of illness, unfitness and poor psycho-social health, though not greatly differentiated by class among young people, were markedly higher in the middle and older years. Rates of disease and impairment, however, offer an unexplained anomaly. These ratio were generally high in industrial areas, but not, at all ages below retirement age, higher among manual social classes than non-manual. After the age of 60, however, rates among those who had been manual workers, or their wives, were poorer. This widening of differences between the classes with age might suggest some effect of the specific manual occupations typical of industrial areas, superimposed upon the already disadvantaging effects of the environment.

82

'Rural and resort' areas provide a contrast. This point is made diagrammatically in Figure 5.5. Again, especially for illness among women and disease/disability among both men and women, class differences widened in middle and older age. For most age/sex groups, however, there was little difference between social classes: to live in this environment is equally healthy for non-manual and manual families.

'Cities', wherever situated geographically, demonstrated health that was as poor as that of industrial areas. When different age-groups and social classes were examined, however, cities (including London) and industrial areas provided a contrast: in cities, it was the psycho-social malaise and illness of *non-manual* men and women that was particularly high. Psycho-social health was outstandingly poor among young non-manual men in London (though numbers here are small) and women in the middle age-group of all social classes in cities. Illness was also very high among these women. On the other hand, non-manual men and women tended to be fitter, and except for women over 60 to have less disease, than those in manual classes in cities and London. Thus it appears that while the adverse environments of industrial areas bear more heavily, for the more 'subjective' components of health, upon those whose socio-economic circumstances are poorer, this is not true for the almost equally adverse environments of cities. Here, non-manual men and women are more strongly affected. For the more 'objective' dimensions of disease and fitness, especially among older people, the city environment reinforces socio-economic disadvantage.

'Areas with a high level of local authority housing' are a rather mixed group, containing parts of the Central Belt of Scotland as well as English New Towns. Perhaps for this reason (but also perhaps because of smaller numbers) class and age trends were more irregular. In general, however, good health in non-manual classes was contrasted, especially in middle and older age, with poor health in manual classes. Manual men and women in the middle years in these areas had particularly poor ratios for all the health dimensions.

It can be concluded that the wider environment of the area of residence, and the socio-economic environment of the household, interact in complex ways. In the more favourable areas (high status areas, rural areas), class differences in health were

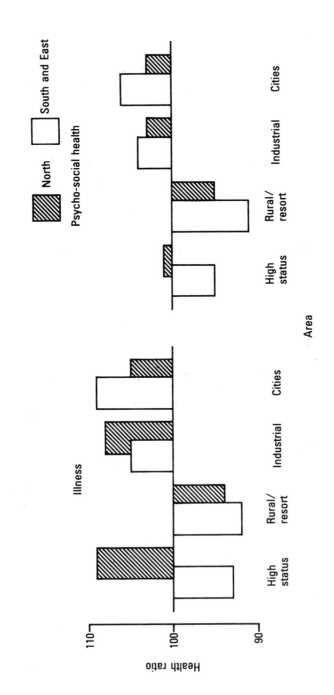

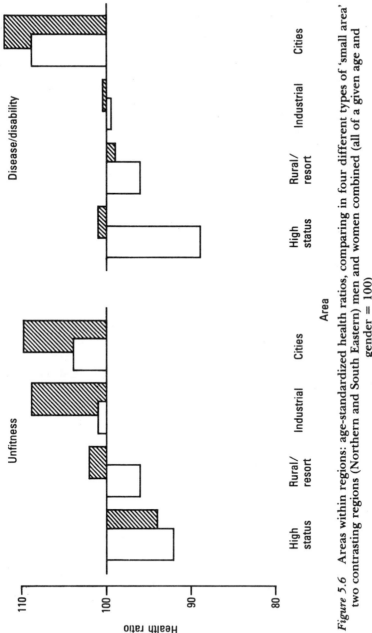

Figure 5.6 Areas within regions: age-standardized health ratios, comparing in four different types of 'small area' two contrasting regions (Northern and South Eastern) men and women combined (all of a given age and gender = 100)

small, at least before old age. This was less true for women than for men, seeming to suggest that women's health is influenced relatively more by 'class' factors, and less by 'environmental' factors. Poor psycho-social health and high illness among young manual-class women in high status areas must be specially noted. In the unfavourable environments of manufacturing and industrial areas, class differences were greater, suggesting that socio-economic and environmental disadvantages have a multiplicative effect. This may also be true in the generally 'unhealthy' environment of cities, but only for the more 'objective' dimensions of health.

Finally, the small area 'families' ought to be considered within geographical regions. Is the disadvantage of the North simply explained by the fact that a high proportion of the older industrial areas are found there? Is the better health of the South and East due wholly to the preponderance of high status residential areas?

Figure 5.6, comparing only the broad regions of the North and the South and East, shows that, in general, the area characteristics represented by the 'families' were more salient than the geographical divisions. As already shown in Figure 5.4, ratios were almost always more favourable in the South and East. If the same types of small area in the geographical region are compared, however, differences between the regions are not great: for illness, psycho-social health and disease in rural or industrial areas they were insignificant, as they were for fitness in family 1. In other words, rural areas were equally healthy, whether in the North or South; 'service centres' showed excess malaise in every part of the country, and indeed rather less in the North than in the South.

A few exceptions may be noted. For each dimension of health except fitness, high status areas in the South and East were more favourable than similar areas in the remainder of the country. The towns and cities of family 4, though always relatively unfavourable to health, were for some components of health less unfavourable in the North than in the South. In fact, it was in the West Midlands, omitted in Figure 5.6, that these cities had the poorest health.

This evidence suggests that the 'North–South divide' has little importance in itself: as the work of Townsend *et al.* mentioned earlier demonstrated, it is the 'local' environment that matters, and there is a greater concentration of poor environments in the North. The 'divide' has significance, if at all, in the best environments. In less favourable types of area, health is very little better in the South.

Unemployment

The unemployed in the Health and Lifestyle Survey have been examined specially, because the relationship between unemployment and health has long been the subject of lively debate (see, e.g. Stern 1983b, Brenner and Mooney 1983, Cook and Shaper 1984, Unemployment and Health Study Group 1986). High mortality rates have been found for unemployed men in, for instance, the OPCS Longitudinal Study (Moser *et al.* 1984) and the British Regional Heart Study (Cook *et al.* 1982), and the General Household Survey has consistently shown higher rates of declared 'long-standing illness' among the unemployed. In 1981–2, for instance, rates for the employed ranging from 7 per cent at age 20–29 to 19 per cent at 50–59 can be compared with rates for the unemployed of 11 per cent at age 20–29 and 33 per cent at age 50–59.

The OPCS Longitudinal Study found particularly high rates for suicide, and many studies have confirmed a relationship between suicide or attempted suicide and unemployment (e.g. Kreitman and Platt 1984, Platt and Kreitman 1984, Hawton and Rose 1986), with the risk increasing with the length of unemployment. Other studies have provided evidence for a deterioration in mental health on becoming unemployed, with improvement if work recommences (Kasl *et al.* 1972, Warr 1984, 1985, Banks and Jackson 1982, Beale and Nethercott 1985).

There are, of course, alternative explanations for these findings. Unemployment may have a direct effect on health through the associated stress and fall in income, and perhaps through changes in behaviour. Alternatively, it can be argued that it is those who are already in poor health who are most likely to become unemployed. Unemployment does not affect all parts of the labour market equally, but is concentrated among semi- and unskilled workers: those who are most vulnerable to ill health are also most vulnerable to unemployment.

However, the OPCS Longitudinal Study, following men who were 'seeking work' at the Census 1971, and controlling for social class, still found excess mortality even though those 'seeking work' were presumed to be in good health (Moser *et al.* 1984). Similar findings related to those 'seeking work' at Census 1981 (Moser *et al.* 1987). In the British Regional Heart Study, the unemployed were divided into those who were 'ill' or 'not ill' at the time they became unemployed, and certain conditions – notably ischaemic heart disease – were raised among both groups. Thus it seems that although some ill health is due to the characteristics of those likely to become unemployed, this cannot altogether account for the excess.

Moreover, the OPCS Longitudinal Study has begun to look at the mortality of other members of households including an unemployed man. The wives of men who were 'seeking work' in 1971 were also found to have raised mortality rates (Moser *et al.* 1986). The children of the unemployed have also been found to have poorer health and development (Maclure and Stewart 1984, MacFarlane and Cole 1985).

The number of unemployed men in the Health and Lifestyle Survey is not very large, and the findings about their health must therefore be treated with caution. (The number of unemployed women is even smaller, and because of the problems associated with defining unemployment in married women, this discussion is confined to unemployed men.) Health ratios, compared with the employed, are shown in Figure 5.7. It should be noted that the health of the employed was slightly better than the average for all men (when age-standardized) because of the effect on the mean of those who are outside the labour market altogether – few in number, but with particularly bad health. Employed men between the ages of 45–59 are shown to have better psycho-social health than the mean, and particularly to have less disease and disability.

The health ratios show that health was poorer for the unemployed at every age and for all the health dimensions. The experience of illness appears to be least associated with unemployment, and the young unemployed were not notably less fit. At all ages psycho-social malaise was higher, however, and particularly high at 30–44. Fitness deteriorated among the unemployed after age 30, and disease/disability were particularly

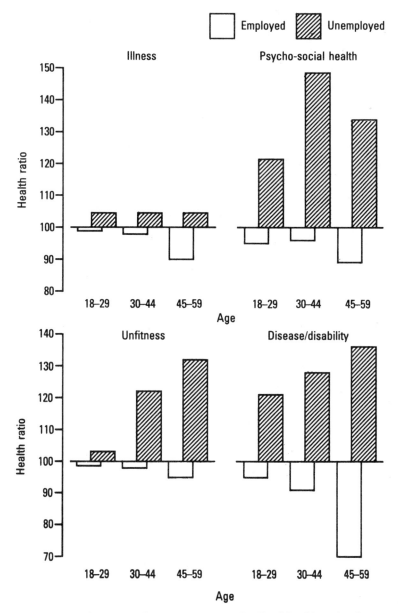

Figure 5.7 Unemployment: age-standardized health ratios for employed and unemployed men age 18–59 (all men of a given age = 100)

high in the later years. It must be emphasized that these men were not the permanently sick, who were defined as out of the labour market rather than unemployed, though it would seem obvious that many of them were, indeed, unemployed because of their sickness.

The numbers of men in higher social classes who are unemployed are too small in this sample to investigate differential class effects reliably. However, the six 'families' of area provide interesting comparisons between unemployment in industrial or rural areas, or suburban or city areas. In industrial and in rural areas, the employed had in fact higher illness ratios than the unemployed (Table 5.6). On the other hand, the illness ratios of the unemployed were particularly unfavourable in high status areas and the towns and cities of family 4. The difference in psycho-social well-being associated with unemployment was also particularly great in family 4, and in industrial areas. In London, however, it was the employed who had high rates of malaise.

Table 5.6   Health ratios for employed and unemployed men aged 18–59 in the six 'families' of area, age-standardized

	Area family					
	1	2	3	4	5	6
	High status	Rural/ resort	Industrial	Cities	L.A. areas	London
Illness						
Employed	94	90	100	100	88	90
Unemployed	108	86	93	115	94	101
Psycho-social health						
Employed	96	82	96	91	100	123
Unemployed	128	114	140	141	136	100
(% unemployed in each area)	(5.5)	(7.4)	(13.4)	(14.1)	(14.4)	(12.6)

Health ratios for the wives of unemployed men were also poorer (Figure 5.8). It is notable here, however, that it appeared to be the younger women who were more affected, and the association of poorer health with an unemployed husband grows weaker with age. After age 45, the psycho-social effect of unemployment appears to bear more heavily upon men than upon their wives.

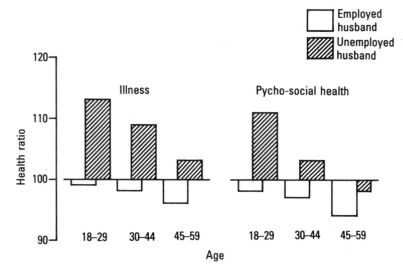

Figure 5.8 Unemployment: age-standardized health ratios, illness and psycho-social health, for the wives of employed and unemployed men (all women of a given age = 100)

To what extent is the 'effect' of unemployment no more than the effect of a low income? Figure 5.9, in which those men, employed or unemployed, with a household income of less than £100/week are singled out, shows that even if employed, those on low incomes had high rates of illness and poor psycho-social health. This is true even at the youngest ages. After the age of 30, however, some additional 'effect' of unemployment is demonstrated: the unemployed were more likely to be unfit and to have long-standing chronic conditions than other men with low incomes. At all ages they were more likely to have poor psycho-social health.

Housing

In considering mortality rates, housing tenure (whether owner-occupied, council rented or other) has been used as a useful surrogate for several dimensions of social class. That is, tenure

91

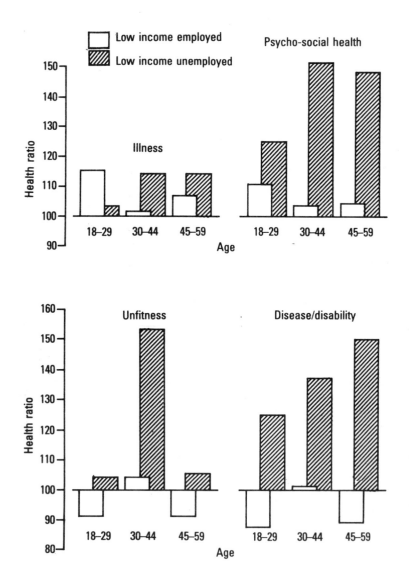

Figure 5.9 Income and unemployment: age-standardized health ratios for men with low household incomes (£100/week or less), comparing the employed and unemployed (all men of a given age = 100)

is assumed to represent not only income, but also capital resources, credit-worthiness, security, and broad standards of housing or the neighbourhood environment. It is not, of course, assumed that these are inevitably superior for every owner-occupier: only that this is a crude division which may tap components of social class other than occupation. It has proved to be a powerful tool for discriminating chances of mortality within social classes (Fox and Goldblatt 1982). Owner occupiers are always shown to have lower mortality than council or other tenants: indeed, there is more variation between owners and tenants within social classes than between social classes within tenure categories.

Table 5.7 shows the proportions of owner-occupiers, council or Housing Association tenants, and others (principally private tenants) in the Health and Lifestyle Survey who were in the broad multi-dimensional categories of 'good/excellent' health, 'poor/very poor' health, and also those in the category of 'good physical health but poor psycho-social health'. It should be noted that it is the tenure of the 'occupier' of the household which is being used here: young people living with owner-occupier parents are put into this category, or elderly people living with a council-tenant child into the category of council tenants. Overall, owner-occupiers are shown to have better health than council tenants, whether they are in non-manual or manual social classes. The difference between owners and tenants was, however, considerably greater for women than for men. For men, there was better health among manual respondents in owner-occupied houses than among non-manual respondents in rented houses. For women, there was a particularly large difference between non-manual respondents in owner-occupied houses and the much poorer health of non-manual respondents in rented accommodation. Indeed, among those in council rented accommodation, women in manual classes were less likely than those in non-manual to be in very poor health, though more likely to be in intermediate health categories – notably the category of poor psycho-social health but good physical health.

The consideration of the health of those in privately-rented and other accommodation is complicated by the fact that a high proportion are young: this is a mixed group, containing both

Table 5.7 Proportions of people by tenure in owner-occupied, council rented, or 'other' housing who are in selected combined health categories

Health category		Owner-occupier		Council tenant		Other	
		Non-man.	Man.	Non-man.	Man.	Non-man.	Man.
		Males					
Good/excellent		39	35	31	28	35	32
Poor/very poor		17	20	25	29	16	27
Good but poor psycho-social health		10	9	10	6	7	10
		Females					
Good/excellent		40	31	20	20	30	31
Poor/very poor		22	23	36	30	21	22
Good but poor psycho-social health		17	18	16	22	21	23
(N = 100%)	M	(1,096)	(1,084)	(165)	(758)	(74)	(98)
	F	(1,305)	(1,186)	(282)	(938)	(105)	(112)

students and others who are likely to have good health, and some families in the very poorest circumstances whose health is likely to be bad. To consider these together is not perhaps very meaningful, but numbers are otherwise small.

The apparently regular trends for the other two tenure categories in Table 5.7 also conceal some interesting differences by age. Amongst men, both the owner-occupier/council tenant differences, and the social class differences, were prominent only in middle years. Among those over 60, council tenants were considerably more likely to have been categorized as having 'poor/very poor' health than owner-occupiers (46 per cent compared with 32 per cent) but there was no difference by social class: the non-manual elderly in council housing had no better health than the manual, and the health of the manual men who own their houses was as good as that of non-manual men.

Among women, as shown in Table 5.8, the particular disadvantage of non-manual women in council housing was shown to apply at every age. The apparent lack of an effect of social class in Table 5.7 upon the proportions of owner-occupiers in poor health is produced by a balancing advantage of younger manual women in owner-occupied houses and disadvantage, compared with non-manual women, as they grow older.

94

Table 5.8 Women at different ages, per cent of different tenure and social class groups in 'good' and 'poor' health categories

	Owner occupier		Council tenant	
	Non-manual	Manual	Non-manual	Manual
Good/excellent health				
Age 18–39	57	44	31	31
40–59	35	31	26	16
60+	23	12	9	13
Poor/very poor health				
Age 18–39	16	12	19	16
40–59	25	28	42	36
60+	37	42	53	48
(N) (18–39)	(527)	(524)	(125)	(378)
(40–59)	(413)	(518)	(70)	(254)
(60+)	(260)	(249)	(87)	(306)

The actual quality of housing – whether it is damp, overcrowded, lacking in amenities or situated in particularly poor local environments – can properly be studied only on a smaller scale, though the use of small area classifications already discussed is relevant. Local studies in recent years relating health specifically to housing conditions include those of Keithley *et al.* (1984) and McCarthy (1985), council housing areas in Gateshead; Department of the Environment (1981), 'difficult to let' council housing in Liverpool; Coleman (1985), flats and houses in London, considering particularly the relationship of housing design to social malaise; Hunt (1986), a deprived area of Edinburgh; Burr *et al.* (1981), in South Wales.

These, and other studies, have particularly associated respiratory symptoms and infections with damp and with ventilation, heating and insulation problems. Likelihood of accidents, particularly among children, and poorer mental health, have been clearly linked to the design of dwellings and of housing schemes.

In the Health and Lifestyle Survey, the information available on housing is not particularly detailed. In Table 5.9 households have, however, been selected on the criteria of (a) overcrowding (more than two persons/bedroom) and (b) lack of amenities (not sole use by the household of kitchen, bathroom, and/or indoor w.c.). These are taken to represent the worst housing conditions.

Virtually no households with high incomes were found in this category, and extremely few non-manual families with an employed breadwinner. There is therefore little point in controlling for social class: the great majority of these households are categorized as classes IV/V. Poor health ratios are notable, especially for the dimension of disease and disability. The rather few (113 individuals) older men and women living in houses which lacked basic amenities were extremely likely to have chronic or disabling conditions, compared with others of the same age. They were not more likely, however, to complain of illness or psycho-social symptoms. Among men, it is in the middle years that exceptionally poor housing was associated with worse health, though among women the association was evident from the youngest years. The majority of the younger men and women in these housing circumstances were married and had children.

Table 5.9 Health ratios for those in housing without amenities and/or crowded housing, standardized for age and gender

	Males			Females		
	Age 18–39	40–59	60+	Age 18–39	40–59	60+
Illness	88	117	97	106	104	98
Psycho-social health	98	107	87	108	109	90
Fitness	106	110	101	113	109	97
Disease/disability	118	137	143	111	117	169
(N)	(220)	(108)	(54)	(288)	(131)	(59)

Households and families

What are the more general associations between household composition and health? Tables 5.10–13 distinguish different life stages. For young people aged 18–29, there was little difference in fitness by household circumstances. Those with more severe disease or disability (relatively few in number) were likely to be living with their parents or others: that is, their health was probably the cause of their living arrangements. Ratios for illness and psycho-social well-being, however, may be assumed to be more likely to be an effect, rather than a cause, of household circumstances. The positive effect of marriage or having a partner on psycho-social well-being is clear. For perceived illness symptoms, it appears that – especially for young single women – living with relatives (usually in the parental home) is very much more favourable than living alone or with others.

Table 5.10   Health ratios for those in different household circumstances, young people 18–29 years, age-standardized

	Illness		Psycho-social health		
	M	F	M	F	(N)
Single, living alone or with other young people	119	134	116	110	(102)
Single, living with relatives (usually parents)	96	93	101	123	(348)
Married or cohabiting, living with partner	98	98	92	94	(266)

In Table 5.11 the extremely disadvantageous effect for women of single-handed parenthood is illustrated, at all ages, especially on psycho-social health. For those women living with a partner, the presence or not of children appeared to make little difference, except that young women without children had less psycho-social malaise.

Table 5.11   Health ratios for women aged 18–45 with and without children, age-standardized

	Illness		Psycho-social health	
	Women aged 18–29	30–45	18–29	30–45
Single parent	125	105	137	142
Married or cohabiting with child(ren)	97	96	99	97
Married or cohabiting without child(ren)	98	95	89	99

It is well known that those who are divorced or separated, or who are widowed in earlier life, or who remain single throughout middle age, tend to have higher mortality than the married (e.g. Berkman and Syme 1979). The explanation may lie in the direct effects of stress, or perhaps different lifestyles, or it may be that selection factors are in operation: those with severe health problems may be less likely to marry, or less likely to remain married because of disorders the spouse cannot tolerate. Since couples share the same environment, poorer life chances may apply to both, and earlier widowhood may be an indicator of this. The widowed and divorced, who had not remarried, of both genders in this survey showed unfavourable health ratios in all the dimensions of health at younger ages, though numbers are relatively small. Those who remained single, however, showed considerably less favourable ratios for men than for women. In the middle years of 40–59 this difference continued: men who were living alone had very much poorer ratios for illness and psycho-social health than women who were living alone. People without a partner who were living with their children – at these ages the children are less likely to be dependent and more likely to be adult – had particularly good ratios for illness, but poor levels of psycho-social health.

Table 5.12   Health ratios for those in different household circumstances aged 45–59, age-standardized

	Illness		Psycho-social health		
	M	F	M	F	(N)
Single, widowed, divorced or separated, living alone	118	96	146	116	(66)
Married or cohabiting, living with partner	99	103	94	92	(656)
Widowed, divorced, or separated, living with own child(ren)	84	82	119	111	(36)

Finally, older people are examined in Table 5.13. Again, there appears to be an interesting difference between men and women. To be still married and living with a spouse was favourable for men's health, but less favourable for women. The healthiest, among women over 60, were those who were widowed but were living with their adult children or other relatives. The men in their 60s living with adult children (though numbers are small) tended to be those without any serious disease or disability, but their illness was high and their psycho-social well-being low. Over 70, widowed men living with their children had relatively poor health on all the dimensions. The generally poorest health, however, was among those (especially men) who lived alone. It is notable that this group of older women was likely to have a high level of disease or disability, compared with those who were not living alone.

Table 5.13   Health ratios for those in different household circumstances, age 60+, age-standardized

	Illness		Psycho-social health		Disease/ disability		(N)
	M	F	M	F	M	F	
Age 60–69							
Living with spouse	98	108	91	94	97	101	(371)
No spouse, living with children or other relatives	108	92	136	88	76	96	(22)
Living alone	114	106	147	114	127	111	(57)
Age 70+							
Living with spouse	92	106	74	91	97	111	(245)
No spouse, living with children or other relatives	111	83	126	82	120	86	(29)
Living alone	120	106	166	113	101	112	(86)

Women, families and employment

Analysis for the unemployed, similar to that for men, is not presented for women. Numbers are lower, which makes results less certain, but the more important issue relates to the meaning of 'employment' for women, especially married women. It is an invariable finding, not only in Britain, that the health of women who are housewives is poorer than that of women who are employed outside the home (Arber 1987). This is true of mortality rates and has been demonstrated for 'long-standing illness' in the General Household Survey. In 1981–2, long-standing illness rates among housewives were higher, except in the youngest years, than among unemployed women. In large part this must be due to those with poorer health choosing not to work outside the home. Formal registration as unemployed is, for married women, very much a function of age or eligibility for benefits: the 'unemployed' do not necessarily represent all those who might choose to work if they could obtain jobs.

Married women's family circumstances, and their health, are therefore an important determinant of whether or not they work outside the home. On the other hand, there is much interest in the effects upon health – particularly mental health – especially if a woman's responsibilities also include the care of children. To be isolated at home with young children can be a cause of stress and depression (Brown and Harris 1978), and the companionship, contribution to self-esteem, and perhaps financial benefits of employment can be positive contributions to health. On the other hand, the 'role strain' of double responsibilities, and the undoubted double work-load within the home and outside it, may also be detrimental to health (Arber *et al.* 1985).

Health ratios for married or cohabiting women aged 18–45, completely age-standardized, are shown in Table 5.14, with the 'employed' (full or part-time) and housewives compared. The women are classified, as in non-manual or manual families, by their husband's occupation, since housewives have no occupational classification of their own, and the use of 'previous occupation' – when women might have been occupied only briefly before marriage, at junior types of job – did not seem to reflect accurately the family's current economic status or life-style. In both non-manual and manual families, housewives tended to have poorer health ratios, whether or not they had children. The element of selection out of employment is clearly demonstrated by the very high ratios for the disease/disability dimension of those who had no children, and were not in paid employment. For those housewives who have children, the lack of paid employment may be a more positive choice, and the ratios were not as high – though always poorer than the employed.

In both broad social classes, those with children had more favourable ratios for illness than those without. This is also true for psycho-social health for non-manual women who worked, but among those who were housewives, malaise was greater amongst those without children.

Thus, though interpretation of cross-sectional data such as this is particularly difficult because of the selection factor,

Table 5.14   Health ratios for married women* aged 18–45 in different social classes and family situations, age-standardized

| | Social class | | | |
| | Non-manual | | Manual | |
	With children	Without	With children	Without
Illness				
Employed[+]	83	104	100	106
Housewife	103	119	107	128
Psycho-social health				
Employed[+]	84	94	102	98
Housewife	102	95	110	120
Disease/disability				
Employed[+]	93	88	89	88
Housewife	110	147	94	206
(N)				
(Employed)[+]	(423)	(203)	(536)	(229)
(Housewife)	(305)	(67)	(471)	(102)

* or cohabiting
+ full or part time

there is no evidence here of ill effects of role strain, or the burden of dual responsibilities. For one group, however, it may be different. For the most part, the trends shown in Table 5.14 were similar in direction and magnitude at all ages. There was one exception: the age-standardized ratios for illness and psycho-social malaise, among women in manual families only, conceal an interesting difference between the youngest and those a little older (Figure 5.10). For manual women up to about the age of 30, with children, working was associated with raised illness, compared with those who were not working, and malaise rates were high for both working mothers and housewives. Thus there is a strong contrast between the social classes in this age-group: for those who had children, working outside the home was favourable for non-manual women, but unfavourable for manual women. Since it is the dimensions of illness and psycho-social health which are involved, and not the more objective dimension of disease, it seems justifiable to impute a causal link: if one's job is pleasant, and perhaps better paid, and resources are more likely to be available for child care, then being a working mother has no ill effects on health; indeed, to be

101

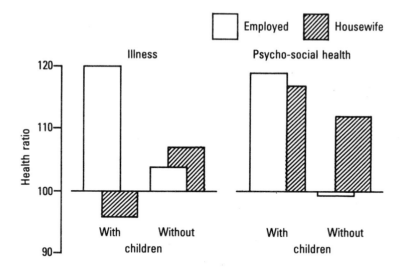

Figure 5.10 Employment of young women with children: age-standardized health ratios, illness and psycho-social health, for married women in manual social classes ages 18–29, with dependent children and without, comparing those who were or were not employed outside the home (all women of a given age = 100)

prevented from working may involve greater stress. If, on the other hand, the job is less pleasant and undertaken principally because of need for money, then dual responsibilities take their toll. These are, of course, generalizations which will not apply to all individuals. Some mechanisms such as this, however, may be prevalent enough to account for the differences by social class in the effects of women's employment.

Social support and social roles

There is much evidence that variables which are more 'social' or personal than socio-economic – social support, integration or isolation, social networks, social roles and activities – are closely associated with health. In a large-scale survey such as this, meaningful information on these topics may not be easy to obtain, and there are also some conceptual problems. These characteristics are even more problematic with regard to the direction of causation than the socio-economic or environmental variables so far discussed. Are people isolated because their mental or physical health is poor, or is the social isolation having an effect on health? If the social contacts of the elderly disabled are frequent, is this because of their special need for help? Or, if they are few, does this demonstrate the problems of the disabled in maintaining social contacts? If people have many community-oriented pursuits and social leisure activities, is this the cause or the result of better health? These questions cannot be answered in a cross-sectional study; they require different kinds of research. Moreover, it is arguable to what extent such characteristics are 'circumstances', presumed to be less voluntary, like the others considered in this chapter, and to what extent they are 'behaviour'. They may represent deliberate choices about particular ways of living: on the other hand they may be ways of life imposed by family, economic, and other personal situations.

Nevertheless, because of the known importance of social support and social integration, some tentative associations in this survey will be demonstrated. In particular, the belief that there is a close relationship between 'stress' and health is a long tradition in our society, as in cultures where the source of illness is seen to lie in troubled social relationships. It will be noted in Chapter 7 that the respondents here not only gave much importance to stress as a cause of ill health in general, thinking that the 'pace and stress' of modern life were important reasons for people being 'less healthy nowadays', but they also cited it as a cause of many specific diseases. Stress, is, of course, not necessarily pathological: it can call up positive responses. But the respondents appeared to be well aware of the increasing evidence that the reaction to prolonged stress can include physiological effects, not only in the specific ways associated with it, e.g. stomach ulcers, but also more generally upon the immune system.

Social loss or social isolation are particular forms of stress which have been shown to be particularly dangerous to health. 'Life events', such as widowhood or other bereavement, divorce, job change, unemployment, migration, even moving from one home to another, are all associated with increased risk of

103

morbidity or mortality (Holmes and Rahe 1967, Sarason *et al.* 1978). The effect of the loss of social relationships is to increase susceptibility to disease (for a review see Totman 1979): there are, however, factors in social life which mediate between potential stressors and vulnerability (Brown and Harris, 1978). Coping mechanisms – strategies and resources for dealing with stress, especially 'chronic' stress – are crucial. Among these is a sense of self-esteem and self-confidence, or the concept defined by Antonovsky (1984) as a 'personal sense of social coherence' which enables people to overcome stress or insulate themselves from stressful environments.

Family relationships and close bonds with intimate friends have been shown to be strongly protective, perhaps through effects on self-esteem and feelings of control (Cobb 1976, Cassel 1976, Heady *et al.* 1985, Pearlin and Schooler 1978) or perhaps through practical consequences relating to health and illness behaviour (Langlie 1977, Scambler *et al.* 1981). Certainly, the relationship between social networks and health has been found to be so strong that it can be used predictively in relation to mortality (Berkman and Syme 1979, House *et al.* 1982), even if risk factors such as smoking are taken into account.

Any direct measurement of stress in this survey presents problems. The respondents were asked if they felt (ever, sometimes or often) under so much stress 'that your health is likely to suffer'. But, since a subjective lack of well-being is one of the measures of health, there is considerable danger of circularity of argument in examining the association of this crude measure of stress with health. It is not surprising that the ratios for the dimension of psycho-social well-being were extremely poor, for all gender, age and social class groups, for those who say that they are 'often' under stress. The relationship of this with other dimensions of ill health may, however, be of interest. Self-perceived stress was strongly associated with poorer health of every kind, but it is notable that the relationship was particularly strong for men in manual classes, at all ages (illness ratios, age-standardized, of 176 for those 'often' under stress, and 128 for those 'sometimes' under stress). The relationship with disease was strong for both men and women and for all classes, but (except, again, for particularly high rates among manual men in middle years) stronger for the young and growing weaker among older age groups. This would seem to be an effect of the greater 'normality' of disease at older ages. Because of the association between disease and fitness, feelings of stress were also associated with lower rates of fitness. It is notable, however, that although the association of stress and disease was of similar magnitude in all social classes, the association of stress and fitness was much stronger, for men but not women, in non-manual than in manual classes. Explanations for this can be no more than speculative. It was noted in Chapter 3 that 'stress' as a cause of ill health in one's life was given greater importance, especially among men, among those in non-manual social classes than among those in manual classes. It seems possible that those non-manual men who knew themselves to be unfit, seeking a reason or an 'excuse', may have been more likely to answer positively to the question about feeling under stress.

Measures of social integration which are available in the Health and Lifestyle Survey may, however, be more informative than this measure of 'stress'. Social integration may be defined objectively, contrasting those who have many social roles and social ties with those who appear to be isolated. Alternatively, subjective feelings about social support may be considered to be more important, whatever the actual family or social situation.

The more objective measure used here is a score of social integration based on a large number of items: household and family situation, frequency of contact with family outside the household and with friends, working status, having children, having surviving parents, whether born in the area, length of residence in the area, attendance at a place of worship, involvement in community work, and whether the individual says that they feel 'part of the community' (Appendix B). This scale represents the number of roles available to the individual, as spouse, child, parent, worker, church member, and so on, combined with some indication of social networks and place in the community. It cannot be regarded as a linear score, but if it is used to categorize people into 'very low', 'low', 'average', 'high' and 'very high' integration groups, there was a strong association of high integration with good health (Figure 5.11). Psycho-social health, in particular, showed a marked decline, for both men and women and in all social classes, as social integration declined: those who had the fewest family, friendship,

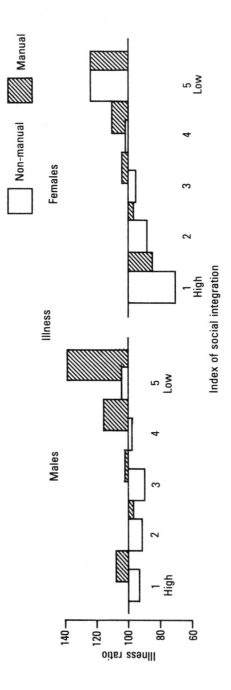

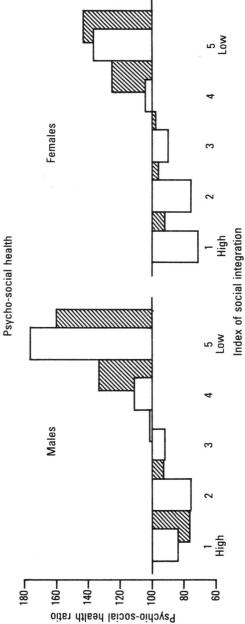

Psycho-social health

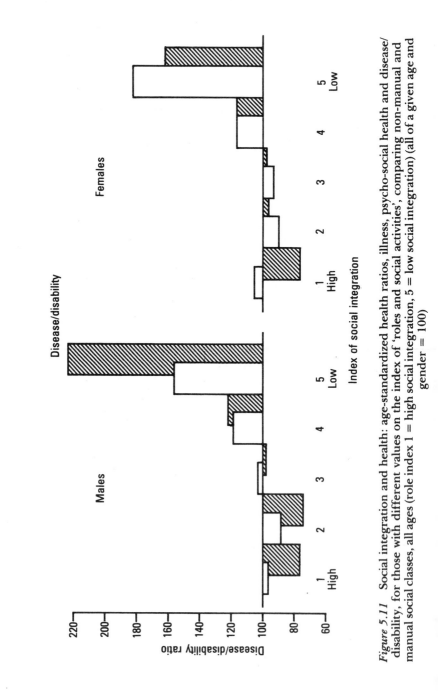

Figure 5.11 Social integration and health: age-standardized health ratios, illness, psycho-social health and disease/disability, for those with different values on the index of 'roles and social activities', comparing non-manual and manual social classes, all ages (role index 1 = high social integration, 5 = low social integration) (all of a given age and gender = 100)

working and community roles had the lowest psycho-social well-being.

There may be some suggestion that 'role overload' may increase illness amongst those with very high scores, among men but not women. This rise in men's illness ratios is accounted for entirely by men in the middle years, among whom the highest integration scores were accompanied by marked rises in illness ratios. Similarly, for non-manual men only, symptoms of psycho-social ill health rose slightly amongst those with the highest scores. It can be noted that there was no evidence of any stress associated with multiple roles (e.g. as mother, worker, socially active) among women.

Some assumption has been made that social integration at least to some extent affects health. It may well be that health affects integration: those who frequently feel themselves to be ill or depressed cut down their social activities. For the dimensions of fitness and disease/disability, it seems likely that it is the individual's health status which is largely dictating activity. Those with chronic disease are, for instance, less likely to be working, and the elderly (who are more likely to have chronic conditions) are more likely than those in middle years to be living alone. Among those over 60, where a higher level of disease is more 'normal', the trends by social integration were less steep than the all-age ratios of Figure 5.11. Nevertheless, it remains true that the most isolated older people tended to be those with the highest level of disease and disability. Among younger people, the highest rate of integration was associated with a rising level of disease and disability, perhaps indicating that their need for family care was being met. (It must be remembered that the survey includes only those people living in the community, and excludes those in any form of residential care.) Considering contact with family outside the household, and with friends, separately as single measures, those men with high levels of contact with family, and to a lesser extent with friends, were those with the highest disease ratios before the age of 60, but the lowest ratios after 60. For women, however, this was less clearly demonstrated.

The subjective measure of social support was based on a simple instrument of seven questions about relationships with family or friends (Appendix B). Degrees of a felt lack of

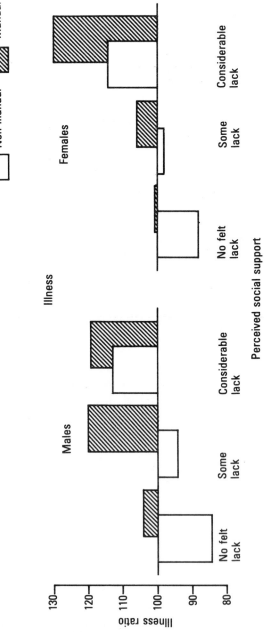

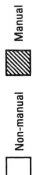

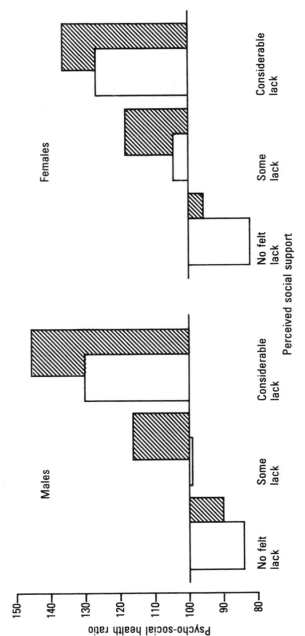

Figure 5.12. Social support and health: age-standardized health ratios, illness and psycho-social health, according to perceived social support, comparing non-manual and manual social classes, all ages (all of a given age and gender = 100)

personal support were related to illness and to psycho-social support in a very regular way (Figure 5.12). Malaise was, as might be expected, affected to a greater extent than illness. It is perhaps of interest to note that women were not more affected by their felt level of emotional support than men, despite a stereotype of the greater importance of emotional factors for women. (That social support is, in fact, less salient for the health of women has been found before however, e.g. House *et al.* 1982). Fitness and disease showed little relationship to perceived social support.

The trends shown in Figure 5.12 were similar for all age-groups, except that at ages over 60, for both men and women, the major distinction appeared to be between a considerable lack of social support and some lack or no lack: it is only when very low social support scores were reached that there was any notable difference in illness or malaise. Amongst those under 60, however, any lack of social support – i.e. anything below the optimum score – raised illness and malaise ratios.

Conclusion

Many of the associations between social circumstances and health are already well known. This analysis, however, has pointed to particular *dimensions* of ill health to which particular groups appear to be vulnerable, and has demonstrated what the protective mechanisms may be – not only resources such as income or a favourable environment, but also personal and social resources such as feelings of social support and integration.

To show that social and economic resources are importantly related to health says nothing, of course, about the way in which these factors operate. To what extent is the effect of low income, or manual social class, or lack of social support, a direct one, and to what extent is it associated with 'unhealthy' behaviour? Patterns of behaviour are the next topic to be considered.

Chapter Six

PATTERNS OF BEHAVIOUR

If the social activities and relationships dealt with in the previous chapter are considered as occupying an intermediate place between 'circumstances' and 'behaviour', four areas of life remain which were specially considered in the Survey. Smoking, the consumption of alcohol, exercise, and diet, were chosen for detailed enquiry because they are the elements of lifestyle usually thought of as most clearly 'voluntary', and undoubtedly associated with health. There can, of course, be debate about the extent to which any of these is always and truly voluntary. Diet may be determined at least in part by income and by the availability of different foods. Smoking and alcohol consumption, in particular, may be regarded less as personal habits than as cultural norms, determined by social pressures. Particular individuals – heavy manual labourers, for instance, or working housewives – may not have the energy or the time to engage in leisure sporting activities. Nevertheless, these four are the lifestyle habits most commonly seen as, at least to some extent, the individual's own responsibility: a 'healthy lifestyle', as currently promulgated, inevitably involves them.

In addition to these four principal habits, two other characteristics are examined, though the status of each as 'behaviour' is rather more problematic. These are overweight or obesity, and sleep patterns. Though each is obviously associated with health, it is of course not possible to claim that either always represents voluntary behaviour. However, the maintenance of normal body weight, and the habit of regular 'approved' hours of sleep, are two of the seven health habits found in the Alameda County Survey (Belloc and Breslow 1972) to correlate with morbidity

113

and predict mortality. They are therefore examined, although more briefly than smoking, alcohol consumption, exercise, and diet.

It has been noted that the behaviours examined here are not the only actions which people can take which are relevant to health. Notable omissions from this survey are data on preventive behaviour, e.g. the taking of dietary supplements, dental hygiene, breast self-examination, the use of car seat-belts; service-use behaviour, both preventive and curative, e.g. the use of check-ups and screening services, the use of medical services when ill; and risk-taking behaviour, e.g. participation in dangerous sports or risky work practices, reckless styles of car driving or motor-cycle riding.

Ideally, of course, one would like information on all these, though the problems of analysis would be formidable. There is considerable evidence that these different sorts of health behaviour do not necessarily make up a consistent set, and that people who engage in one cannot be reliably predicted to engage in another (Mechanic 1979, Steele and McBroom 1972, Calnan 1985). In the present analysis, the four major habits examined have to 'stand in' for a general concept of healthy or unhealthy lifestyle. The assumption is that an individual who smokes and drinks heavily, and is careless of the health implications of exercise and diet, is leading a generally unhealthy life, for which other forms of health behaviour such as the use of preventive services is unlikely to compensate.

THE FOUR BEHAVIOURS

For each of the four areas of behaviour, simple scales with six levels were formed (Appendix C). Their derivation, and probable reliability, are discussed below. They are considered only as categories ranked from 'good' to 'bad', and not as interval scales.

There is no intention of offering here a detailed description of the patterning of individual items of behaviour in this sample of the population at the time of the survey (see Cox *et al.* 1987). Such information quickly goes out of date. Moreover, better data on each specific topic, for instance on diet or alcohol consumption, is available from specialized surveys which a wide-ranging enquiry such as this could not hope to match. The special feature of the data here is the possibility of examining overall lifestyles, and asking, 'Do unhealthy behaviours substitute for one another, or cluster and reinforce each other? To what extent are patterns of behaviour associated with health?'

Smoking

A scale representing the amount of smoking, ranging from 'non-smoker' to 'heavy smoker' (20+ cigarettes/day) is easy to form, and the distribution of smoking habits in different age/gender groups is shown in Table 6.1. The only problematic issue is whether ex-smokers should be given a special rank. (This point is also relevant to alcohol consumption.) Since this is a survey of behaviour and health at one moment of time, it was decided that it was not justifiable to include previous behaviour. A wide range of patterns involving the level of previous smoking or alcohol consumption and the time since giving up would have to be accommodated: nor, in any case, is any change in behaviour available for diet and exercise. This is not to say, of course, that previous smoking patterns are irrelevant to health: merely that ex-smokers have to be considered separately.

Table 6.1 Distribution of smoking categories, per cent

| Category* | Males | | | | Females | | | |
	Age 18–39	40–59	60+	All	Age 18–39	40–59	60+	All
(Current) non-smoker	53	50	56	53	62	62	74	65
Pipe or cigar smoker	6	11	14	9	1	1	1	1
Occasional cigarette smoker	3	2	1	2	2	2	1	2
Light regular cigarette smoker	11	8	10	10	12	12	12	12
Moderate regular cigarette smoker	21	18	14	19	19	18	11	17
Heavy regular cigarette smoker	6	10	5	7	4	4	1	3

* See Appendix C

The reliability of the data obtained on smoking can be assessed only by comparison with other national surveys, especially those specifically focused on smoking and thus likely to be more detailed. By these standards, it appears that the smoking information is generally accurate. The prevalence of regular cigarette smoking (defined as more than one cigarette per day) was 36 per cent of men and 32 per cent of women. This can be compared with rates of 38 per cent and 33 per cent found by Marsh and Matheson (1983), and similar figures in the General Household Survey of 1982.

The slightly lower smoking rate in this survey may reflect a continuing decline in smoking: the comparable rates in 1972 were 53 per cent for men and 41 per cent for women (GHS 1972). This decline is due more to existing smokers giving up than to young people avoiding the habit. In 1972 19 per cent of the population declared themselves as ex-smokers, compared with 27 per cent (men) and 20 per cent (women) claiming to be ex-regular smokers in this survey. As in other surveys, the most common age at which current smokers said that they started to smoke was in adolescent years, 14 for men and 16 for women.

Smoking is strongly associated with education and with social class (Table 6.2). The decline has been rather steeper among men than among women, and considerably steeper among those in non-manual social classes than among manual workers and their wives. Thus a narrowing differential between men and women has gone hand in hand with a widening social class difference. In this survey, as in others, there is now little difference in regular cigarette smoking between men and women in non-manual social classes, but a considerable difference in semi-skilled and unskilled families.

Table 6.2 Smoking in different socio-economic groups, per cent

	Profes-sional	Employers/ managers	Other non-man.	Skilled man.	Semi-skilled	Un-skilled
Males						
Always non-smokers	34	25	31	22	21	17
Ex-smokers	29	30	26	27	25	22
Regular cigarette smokers	17	28	26	38	45	50
Other*	20	17	17	13	9	10
(N)	(188)	(695)	(685)	(1,402)	(647)	(210)
Females						
Always non-smokers	52	49	53	43	42	32
Ex-smokers	30	21	19	19	18	19
Regular cigarette smokers	14	28	26	35	37	45
Other*	6	2	3	3	3	4
(N)	(262)	(867)	(1,160)	(1,607)	(845)	(233)

* Occasional cigarette smokers, pipe and cigar smokers, unclassifiable

116

Smoking prevalence also varies between geographical regions (in part because of occupational distributions), with the highest rates in Scotland and the North West, and the lowest in the South East. More interestingly, however, examination of the small area 'families' used in Chapter 5 shows that class is related to smoking in different ways in different types of area. Some examples are shown in Table 6.3. Smoking prevalence was generally high in cities, including London, and in traditional industrial areas. There was little difference, among men, between non-manual and manual classes in rural or resort and retirement areas. Among women, a strong class difference remained in these areas, and smoking among women in resort/retirement areas was generally high. For both men and women, the class difference was most marked in the family of 'areas with high local authority housing'.

Table 6.3 Percentages of smokers (any smoking) in different 'families' of area, comparing non-manual and manual social classes, all ages <60

Area family	*Males*		*Females*	
	Non-man.	*Man.*	*Non-man.*	*Man.*
High status	39	52	31	38
Rural	45	50	22	38
Resort/retirement	40	38	34	51
Industrial	49	62	31	49
L.A. housing	38	54	28	53
Cities, London	48	58	34	53
(N = 100%)	(349)	(343)	(475)	(372)
	(165)	(208)	(246)	(279)
	(77)	(87)	(122)	(104)
	(269)	(537)	(405)	(651)
	(97)	(160)	(139)	(166)
	(232)	(342)	(334)	(399)

Alcohol consumption

Alcohol consumption was measured by asking the respondents whether they drank, and if so whether only on special occasions or more regularly; by enquiry about past drinking; and by a seven-day diary method taking them through their drinking 'last week'. The diary method is usually considered to be the best available for producing reliable information (Pernanen 1974), and the mean amounts declared were very close indeed to those reported in specialized national studies of alcohol consumption (Wilson 1980, Dight 1976). The distribution of different categories of drinking by age and gender is shown in Table 6.4, where the categorization of light, moderate and heavy drinking is based on the standard definitions used in these surveys.

Table 6.4 Distribution of categories of alcohol consumption, per cent

Category*	Males				Females			
	Age 18–39	40–59	60+	All	18–39	40–49	60+	All
Non-drinker	5	6	11	6	8	12	22	12
Very occasional drinker	7	12	21	11	20	22	34	24
Regular drinker, none 'last week'	9	11	10	10	17	12	8	14
Light drinker	26	28	25	29	27	28	22	26
Moderate drinker	46	38	16	39	28	25	13	24
Heavy drinker	8	5	3	6	1	1	1	1

*See Appendix C

A few questions were asked to apply a standard brief screening test for problem drinkers or those with a dependence on alcohol. It seems, however, that those with a very heavy consumption or an alcohol 'problem' were, not surprisingly, underrepresented in the survey or less likely to report their drinking accurately, since the rate is less than the prevalences usually estimated or found in specialized surveys (Royal College of Psychiatrists 1978). Thus the health consequences of heavy, dependent drinking are not a topic which can be accurately dealt with. This is a relatively small and well-studied group, however, and perhaps of less importance in an analysis which seeks to consider typical, 'ordinary', behaviour patterns rather than the already well-known effects of extreme health-harming behaviour.

The distribution of drinking habits declared in the survey showed commonly-demonstrated patterns: not only the heavier drinking of men, especially young men, and greater likelihood of non-drinking among women, especially older women, which are demonstrated in Table 6.4, but also regional and social differences. The average number of units of alcohol consumed 'last week', among those who drank at all, was highest among men in the North (26.5 units) and lowest in East Anglia (14.4 units). Women's average consumption, though always much less than men's, was on the other hand comparatively low in the North and Scotland and highest in Greater London. The North also displayed the highest proportion of male ex-drinkers (10 per cent of all men), and Scotland the highest proportion of both male and female non-drinkers.

Again, however, the use of 'small areas' modified these generalizations. Wherever they were situated geographically, more moderate/heavy drinking was recorded in traditional industrial and manufacturing areas (Table 6.5). In these areas, there were higher rates of moderate/heavy drinking among men (but not women) in manual social classes, compared with non-manual. In 'high status' areas, however, and in London, non-manual men were the more frequent heavy drinkers. Thus the relationship of social class to drinking habits depends very much on the environment: statements about relative social class consumption are not wholly straightforward.

Table 6.5 Percentages in different 'families' of area who are moderate/heavy drinkers, comparing non-manual and manual classes, all ages <60

Area family	Males		Females	
	Non-man.	Man.	Non-man.	Man.
High status	50	44	30	32
Industrial	49	58	36	32
L.A. housing	40	49	25	22
London	52	45	36	21
(N = 100%)	(349)	(343)	(475)	(372)
	(269)	(537)	(405)	(651)
	(97)	(160)	(139)	(166)
	(87)	(72)	(114)	(82)

At least moderate drinking was most common among men in the employer/manager, own-account trades, and skilled manual occupational categories at younger ages, and among professionals as well as employers and managers in the middle years. The retired drank less, and the unemployed were more likely not to drink than the employed (though not less likely, among

119

those who did drink, to have a heavy consumption). Women working outside the home were more likely to drink than housewives, and women in non-manual families more likely than those in manual families. Beer drinkers, and those who drank both beer and spirits, were likely to have the highest consumption.

Exercise

Exercise is defined solely as leisure-time physical activity. It is generally agreed that this is what is relevant to health, especially

Table 6.6   Distribution of exercise categories, per cent, comparing non-manual and manual social classes

Category*	Age 18–39		40–59		60+	
	Non-man.	Man.	Non-man.	Man.	Non-man.	Man.
Males						
1 High level of vigorous exercise	25	22	14	9	7	4
2 Moderate level of vigorous exercise	23	18	15	10	6	6
3 Some vigorous exercise	17	11	10	9	7	6
4 Some exercise but no sports, keep-fit etc.	9	13	16	15	17	19
5 Little exercise	9	13	21	29	31	27
6 No exercise	17	22	25	28	32	36
(N = 100%)	(673)	(953)	(516)	(724)	(362)	(630)
Females						
1 High level of vigorous exercise	14	9	9	7	3	2
2 Moderate level of vigorous exercise	21	15	13	10	4	7
3 Some vigorous exercise	19	16	16	12	7	4
4 Some exercise but no sports, keep-fit, etc.	13	16	13	13	12	13
5 Little exercise	15	21	21	26	27	24
6 No exercise	19	23	29	33	47	51
(N = 100%)	(994)	(1,119)	(727)	(852)	(515)	(806)

* See Appendix C

for protection against coronary heart disease, and activity which is undertaken as part of work is a matter which has to be considered separately (Morris *et al.* 1980). Respondents to the survey were asked in detail about the sporting and other energetic activities, including keep-fit activities, which they had done 'in the last fortnight', and also about the time spent in leisure-time walking and gardening. The scale used in Table 6.6 is derived from calculations of the energy expended in all these activities. The possibility arises, of course, that 'the last fortnight', may not represent a typical period for some individual respondents. However, the patterns of activity which resulted appeared to have a good face validity, and this form of questioning was thought preferable to more general and less quantifiable descriptions.

Leisure-time physical activity is, of course, strongly related to age. Among men under 40, 17 per cent claimed to have done some running or jogging in 'the last fortnight', and 20 per cent of women of the same age said that they had engaged in some keep-fit activity. Only 3 per cent of women over 60 did so. The more active sporting pursuits and keep-fit activities were also, among those under 60, much more likely to be part of the lifestyle of those with higher educational qualifications and those in non-manual rather than manual households. For instance, among those aged 18–40 years, 42 per cent (male) and 51 per cent (female) in manual households said that they took part in no sporting or keep-fit activities at all, although they might have done some walking or gardening, compared with 30 per cent (male) and 38 per cent (female) in non-manual households. This pattern of participation matches well with that which has been reported in other surveys of the British population (e.g. General Household Survey 1978).

In different areas of residence, the social class patterns of men and women over 60 did not greatly differ. Amongst younger people, however, traditional industrial areas were notable not only because smaller proportions overall declared a 'good' rate of exercise, but also because there was little difference between social classes (and indeed a reversed trend among men in middle age) (Table 6.7). In cities and service centres, including London, there were high rates of vigorous exercise, perhaps representing the availability of sporting facilities. In these areas, however, non-manual men and women were considerably more likely than manual to describe a high level of exercise. In rural areas, and in 'high status' areas, class differences were small among young men, but considerable among men in the middle years and women of all ages.

Table 6.7 Percentages in different 'families' of area with high levels of exercise comparing non-manual and manual social classes, age <60

Area families		Age 18–39		40–59	
		Non-man.	Man.	Non-man.	Man.
		Males			
High status		45	41	30	19
Rural		44	42	27	17
Industrial		38	35	17	21
Cities, London		51	41	28	20
		Females			
High status		36	25	20	14
Rural		37	22	27	16
Industrial		30	30	18	13
Cities, London		40	22	20	15
(N = 100%)	(M)	(200)	(189)	(149)	(154)
		(75)	(114)	(90)	(94)
		(162)	(331)	(107)	(206)
		(138)	(178)	(94)	(164)
	(F)	(290)	(211)	(185)	(161)
		(119)	(152)	(127)	(127)
		(227)	(385)	(178)	(266)
		(215)	(213)	(119)	(186)

Diet

The development of an index of good/bad diet presented problems. The survey did not include measured quantities of food intake, but only a more qualitative description of the 'usual' diet, based on a list of foods, with the request to say how often ('more than once a day'/'once a day', 'most days', etc.) they were eaten. In addition, questions were asked about various specific dietary habits – bread eating, what was spread on bread, tea and coffee drinking, etc. There is no measure of the quantity of diet.

Complex derived variables, such as estimations of the total sugar or fat consumption, were examined as candidates for inclusion in an overall index of diet. It was found, however, that the use of simple single variables gave much the same results. Items were selected which would represent dietary habits currently approved by nutritionists, and a discriminant analysis was performed to test their efficiency as predictors of a combination variable. Several items were rejected, either because they added no discrimination or because they did not prove to be associated with an overall 'good' or 'bad' diet. For instance, it was thought that the answers to the questions, 'Do you eat regularly, that is, do you have the same number of meals and snacks at roughly the same time each day?' and 'How many times a day do you have a snack or something to eat between meals?' might be candidates for inclusion, since snack-eating is often said to be a bad dietary habit and regular meals a good one. In fact, neither was consistently associated with diets otherwise characterized as bad. For some age-groups (e.g. females over 60) irregularity of meals was significantly associated with otherwise good diets. It seemed that 'small but frequent' meals might well consist of 'healthy' foodstuffs.

Ultimately, only seven specific food habits from among those available were found to be, together, an efficient indicator of a nutritionally approved diet: eating predominantly wholemeal/brown bread, eating low fat or polyunsaturated spreads, eating fresh fruit at least once a day in summer, eating salads or raw vegetables at least once a week in winter, eating chips not more than twice a week, eating other fried food not more than twice a week, and not eating sweets/biscuits every day.

A 'good' diet, so defined, was more common among women than men. A high proportion of young men, in particular, had very few good dietary habits. The highest scores were most likely amongst women of middle age.

It is well known that diet in Britain is associated with social class and with region. This survey agreed well with e.g. the Household Food Consumption and Expenditure Surveys. Considering individual items of diet, predominantly brown or wholemeal bread rather than white was eaten by 49 per cent of professional families, and by only 17 per cent of unskilled families, and by 43 per cent of those in the South East compared with 21 per cent in the West Midlands (respondents under 50 years). Fruit was eaten rarely or never (in summer) by 38 per cent of over-60s in Wales, and by 12 per cent in the South East. The use of low fat or polyunsaturated spreads was described by 43 per cent of all women in professional families, and 15 per cent in unskilled families (Cox *et al.* 1987).

Table 6.8 compares area 'families', wherever situated geographically. That women were more likely to have 'good' food habits than men, and those in non-manual social classes more likely than those in manual, is shown to be true in every type of area. 'High status' areas, for all age groups, and rural/resort areas, for all women but not older men, were the areas where the best diets were found. Diets were notably poor in areas with high local authority housing. The difference between social classes was remarkably constant in all areas, though in general least in rural/resort areas and greatest in cities, including London. In these city areas relatively high proportions of non-manual men and women had 'healthy' diets – except for elderly men, diets were as good as they were in 'high status' areas. For manual men and women living in cities, however, diets appeared to be likely to be particularly 'unhealthy'.

Table 6.8   Percentage of those in different 'families' of area with good diets, by social class (5+ 'good' food habits)

	Males						Females					
	Age 18–39		40–59		60+		18–39		40–59		60+	
Area family	NM	M	NM	M	NM	M	NM	M	NM	M	NM	M
High status	35	18	45	30	51	30	49	36	59	45	54	39
Rural/resort	39	18	31	24	36	25	53	42	56	41	54	36
Industrial	31	13	35	17	40	17	43	24	52	38	42	37
Cities/London	35	16	44	20	39	16	50	24	55	33	53	30
L.A. Housing	22	10	40	22	–	14	36	21	42	30	–	29
(N = 100%)	(213)	(203)	(154)	(159)	(97)	(133)	(303)	(224)	(193)	(167)	(114)	(164)
	(110)	(156)	(121)	(128)	(118)	(142)	(167)	(209)	(187)	(168)	(171)	(135)
	(150)	(301)	(100)	(198)	(69)	(178)	(212)	(360)	(167)	(253)	(98)	(218)
	(146)	(200)	(98)	(172)	(66)	(125)	(217)	(229)	(127)	(195)	(98)	(203)
	(54)	(93)	(43)	(67)	(12)	(52)	(86)	(97)	(53)	(69)	(36)	(86)

Thus the overall scores were clearly patterned by education, and social class, and region. An important underlying variable associated with all these appeared to be income. Table 6.9 therefore compares those below an arbitrary 'low household income' line with those above. It can be noted that in all age/gender groups – though least for young men – those with low incomes were very much more likely than those with high to have fewer 'good' dietary habits.

Table 6.9   Diet – comparison of those with 'high' and 'low' household incomes (percentage)

Number of 'bad' food habits	Age 18–39		40–59		60+	
	Income High	Low	High	Low	High	Low
	Males					
0–2	10	7	16	7	20	8
3–4	40	28	45	38	49	44
5+	50	65	39	55	31	48
(N = 100%)	(764)	(535)	(602)	(477)	(177)	(666)
	Females					
0–2	23	11	26	18	26	14
3–4	47	41	54	45	56	52
5+	30	48	20	37	17	34
(N = 100%)	(874)	(839)	(581)	(616)	(110)	(956)

It may be, of course, that these apparently strong effects of income are in fact a result of class-related differences in income, or the regional distribution of incomes. All these influences upon diet are clearly inter-related. In order to tease out the relationships, a multivariate (loglinear) analysis was performed, using the variables region, income, and education (to represent the less 'economic' and more 'cultural' aspects of social class). Together, these proved to be good predictors of a good or bad diet. Other things being equal, however, it was education that had the greatest effect, for every age/gender group except women in the mid-age group (Table 6.10). Younger and older women with no educational qualifications were more than twice as likely to have a poor diet, when compared with someone otherwise similar but with educational qualifications. The effect of education was also strong for men, and grew stronger with age. When the other variables were taken into consideration, income, of itself, had a significant effect only for women under 60, and was the most important predictor of poor diet only for women in the middle years: a woman aged 40–59 with a low income was 1.52 times as likely to have a poor diet as one with a high income, other things being equal. Region (defined simply as North/South) retained an important effect for all those under 60. A young man or woman in the North was 1.42 times as likely as one in the South to have a poor diet, other things being equal. For men and women over 60, region of itself had a small, and not significant, *negative* effect: that is, diets were at least as good in the North as in the South, once income and education were allowed for. No interaction effects reached significance in this analysis, except the interaction of region and education for older men: those in the North with low education had poorer diets than the effect of each alone might suggest.

Table 6.10 Odds ratios (loglinear analysis): association of region, income, and education with diet

	Males			Females		
	Age 18–39	40–59	60+	18–39	40–59	60+
Odds on poor diet						
Region – North:South	1.42	1.31	NS	1.42	1.39	NS
Income – low:high	NS	NS	NS	1.24	1.52	NS
Education – no qualifications: qualifications	1.58	1.67	1.78	2.04	1.45	2.37
Interaction of region and education	NS	NS	1.25	NS	NS	NS

Thus is seems that the apparent relationship of income and diet of Table 6.9 is largely an effect of regional differences and the more 'cultural' or educational aspects of social class. For women under 60, however, low income remained an important predictor of a poor diet even when these other factors are controlled for.

Sleep patterns

'Approved' hours of sleep, defined as 7–8 hours, is commonly considered as healthy behaviour. In this survey, the population was almost evenly divided between those who claimed to sleep for 7–8 hours, those who 'usually' slept for less, and those who 'usually' had longer hours. Younger men and women were more likely to quote more than 8 hours; the proportions who slept under 7 hours rose steeply with age.

The question arises, however, as to the extent to which habitual hours of sleep are truly a 'voluntary' behaviour. Obviously, there may be individuals who choose to sleep unusually long or short hours. Various personality factors and psychosocial malaise symptoms were examined as predictors of sleeping habits: those people who said that they were 'under strain' and those who had high neuroticism scores in the Eysenck Personality Inventory (groups who were, of course, likely to overlap) were more likely to claim less than 7 hours sleep. On the other hand, 'worrying', depression, or 'always feeling tired', were not clearly associated with hours of sleep. The overwhelmingly dominant predictor of sleeping habits was the individual's health status. Irrespective of age, those who had no chronic conditions were most likely to sleep for 7–8 hours. At the other extreme, those with moderately or severely handicapping conditions were both more likely to sleep for less than 7 hours or to sleep for more than 8. Twelve per cent of this latter group, among men and women over 40, quoted more than 9 hours sleep (compared with 5 per cent of those with no disease) and 50 per cent claimed less than 7 hours (compared with 37 per cent of those with no disease).

Thus the association of current health and current sleeping habits is so strong that the use of sleeping habits as another 'voluntary' behaviour (in a survey at one moment of time) does not appear to be justified.

Weight control

Another possible contender for inclusion as a 'health behaviour' is weight control. There is no doubt that the avoidance of overweight is important for health, and it is perhaps more clearly within the individual's control than sleep behaviour. Body mass index (weight/height^2) was calculated from the measurements made in this survey, and categories of underweight/acceptable weight/mildly overweight/obese derived (see Cox *et al.* 1987: ch. 4): the prevalence of underweight and of obesity among age and social class groups is shown in Table 6.11. Here again, however, the association of present health status and weight status confuses any consideration of weight control as health behaviour. Those people with chronic disease conditions were very much more likely to be underweight, especially among men over 40. They were also more likely to be obese, especially among women under 60. (It must be remembered that 'obesity' might itself be offered as a chronic condition.) Accounts of attempts to control weight were obtained in the survey, and it is possible that these, together with measured body mass index and perhaps dietary data, might be used to provide an index of this behaviour. However, the timing of events is complex and the validity of the accounts problematic: it was therefore decided that, like sleeping habits, weight control could not be included in this analysis.

Table 6.11 Distribution of body mass index categories by social class, per cent (all ages)

Body mass index category	Social class					
	Professional	Employers/ managers	Other non-man.	Skilled man.	Semi-skilled	Un-skilled
Males						
Underweight	9	5	6	8	10	10
Acceptable weight	52	45	53	49	49	46
Overweight	34	41	35	36	34	31
Obese	5	10	6	9	7	13
Females						
Underweight	3	4	5	5	4	4
Acceptable weight	57	51	56	45	45	43
Overweight	34	31	27	32	35	34
Obese	6	13	12	18	17	19

ASSOCIATION OF THE FOUR BEHAVIOURS

So far, smoking, alcohol consumption, exercise and diet have been considered separately. To what extent are the four 'unhealthy' behaviours linked in individuals? Rather little information on general patterns has previously been available. It is well-known that smoking and alcohol consumption are associated (Wilson 1980, Dight 1976), with non-drinkers more likely to be non-smokers. The British Regional Heart Study (O'Cummins *et al.* 1981) found that among men aged 40–59, 'frequent light drinkers' were least likely to be heavy or moderate smokers, and heavy daily drinking was associated with heavy smoking. It is also known that very heavy alcohol consumption – at a level which is associated with alcohol-related disease or dependence – is likely to be accompanied by a poor diet. These known associations apart, however, any apparent connection between these aspects of behaviour rests only on the fact that each varies by social class, or education, or region.

There is a stereotype of the individual who leads a positively healthy lifestyle – a committed non-smoker, and at most a light drinker, who actively engages in keep-fit activities, goes jogging, or plays sports, and carefully chooses a low-fat, low-sugar, high-fibre, 'natural' diet. At the other extreme, there is an image of the person who is wholly careless of their health, at whom the health educators' messages are principally directed. He or she – though the stereotype is perhaps more often male – is likely to be pictured at the extremes of the social scale: the over-eating, over-drinking, sedentary expense-account life, or the heavy smoking and drinking, poor diet and lack of sports or keep-fit activities felt to be associated with poverty or unemployment in deprived Northern urban areas.

To what extent do these people really exist, or what proportion of the population do they represent? To answer this it is necessary to consider the inter-relation of the four behaviours, so that – in subsequent chapters – the purposive or otherwise nature of overall lifestyles can be examined, and the cumulative effects on health investigated.

The correlation of the four indices of behaviour (Spearman's rank order correlation) is shown in Table 6.12. Because of the nature of the indices, these can be regarded as no more than indications of the relative strength of associations between the four habits, but they are a first step towards the consideration of overall behaviour patterns. Which of these four aspects of lifestyle are most likely to vary together, and do the associations differ by social class?

Table 6.12 Correlation (Spearman's *rho*) of indices of exercise, diet, smoking, alcohol consumption, in different age and gender groups

In each case three age-groups are shown separately: younger (18–39), mid (40–59), older (60+)

		Males Non-manual			Manual		
		Exercise	Smoking	Diet	Exercise	Smoking	Diet
Smoking	(Y)	0.02			0.18**		
	(M)	0.02			0.13**		
	(O)	0.06			0.02		
Diet	(Y)	0.05	0.13**		0.11**	0.16**	
	(M)	0.02	0.24**		0.08*	0.24**	
	(O)	0.11*	0.29**		0.12**	0.21**	
Alcohol	(Y)	−0.05	0.12**	0.10*	0.02	0.13**	0.10**
	(M)	−0.07	0.17**	0.03	0.03	0.15**	0.10**
	(O)	−0.12*	0.08	0.03	0.14**	0.09*	0.05
		Females Non-manual			Manual		
Smoking	(Y)	0.00			0.04		
	(M)	0.01			0.06		
	(O)	−0.02			−0.04		
Diet	(Y)	0.13**	0.17**		0.10**	0.22**	
	(M)	0.11*	0.19**		0.13**	0.23**	
	(O)	0.14**	0.17**		0.17**	0.16**	
Alcohol	(Y)	−0.05	0.17**	0.01	−0.12**	0.13**	−0.02
	(M)	−0.10*	0.14**	−0.04	−0.17**	0.07	−0.06
	(O)	−0.07	0.12**	−0.05	−0.10*	0.08*	−0.08

* $p<.01$; ** $p<.001$

It is obvious that smoking and diet are the most highly correlated, for both genders and at all ages. Those who smoke were likely to have a poor diet, and those who do not smoke a better one. This association has been investigated in more detail in the Health and Lifestyle sample by Whichelow *et al.* (1988).

Smoking and alcohol consumption are also associated, though less strongly. It should be noted here that ex-drinkers, credited with 'healthy' behaviour on the drinking index, were in fact the most likely of all the categories of drinker to be heavy smokers. The association of diet and alcohol consumption is interestingly different for men and for women. For men, drinking was correlated with a poor diet, though weakly in both broad social classes. For women, in contrast, drinking was consistently though weakly associated with a good diet.

Alcohol consumption is also consistently associated, for non-manual men and all women, with a *high* level of exercise. Among women, the association is stronger in manual than non-manual classes: those with the highest consumption, especially under 60, were likely to take the most exercise, and non-drinkers were more likely to have poor exercise habits. Among men, there were strong correlations only for those over 60: elderly men in non-manual classes were more likely to associate good levels of exercise with higher levels of alcohol consumption, while men in manual classes were likely to drink *less* if their exercise level was high.

Finally, exercise and diet again show a difference between women and men. For women, irrespective of social class, a good diet and a high level of exercise were strongly correlated. Among men there was a strong association only in manual classes.

In general, the association between different habits is strongest for young men in manual classes. For this group, all behaviours except alcohol consumption were correlated: those with one 'unhealthy' habit were likely to have others, and 'healthy' lifestyles were likely to be consistent. Non-manual men had the least likelihood of consistently 'healthy' or 'unhealthy' behaviour.

PATTERNS OF BEHAVIOUR

How, then, do these four behaviours combine in individuals? In order to provide a clear description, simplified categories are necessary. In Figures 6.1–3, a primary distinction is made between smoking and non-smoking, here counting as 'smokers' all those who smoke at all, whatever their consumption, and

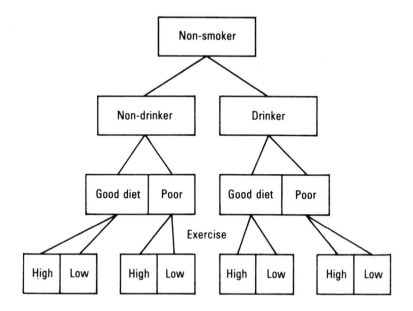

Percentage of different age/gender groups following pathway

Males

18–39	11	4	9	5	9	2	10	4
40–59	10	11	5	7	5	5	4	3
60+	11	18	5	11	4	4	2	3

Females

18–39	21	12	8	8	7	2	3	2
40–59	18	20	4	8	7	4	1	1
60+	12	35	3	16	3	5	1	2

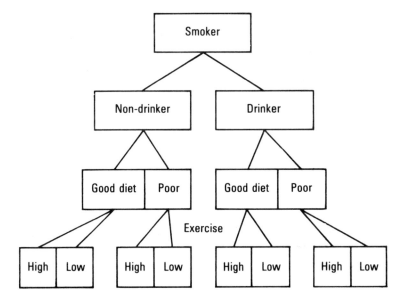

Percentage of different age/gender groups following pathway

5	3		7	4		6	2		12	7
6	6		5	9		5	4		7	8
5	8		5	11		2	2		2	5
8	4		6	6		5	2		4	2
6	9		4	8		4	3		1	2
3	8		2	6		1	1		1	1

Figure 6.1 Combinations of different 'healthy' and 'unhealthy' behaviours, showing the percentages of each age/gender group displaying each combination

including cigar and pipe smokers. Alcohol consumption, on the other hand, is considered as perhaps 'unhealthy' behaviour only if it is at least 'moderate' (categories 5 and 6 in the alcohol consumption scale) since there is no evidence that occasional or light drinking is harmful to health. Exercise is divided into arbitrary categories of high (some vigorous exercise, categories 1–3), and low (no vigorous exercise, categories 4–6); diet into categories of good (5+ good food habits) and poor (4 or fewer good food habits).

Figure 6.1 shows the possible 'pathways', or combinations, with the proportions of different age/gender groups who displayed each behaviour pattern. A notable point is how varied patterns of behaviour are, even in this very simplified model. It is certainly not true that the population can be easily divided into those who lead healthy lifestyles, and those who do not: most people's patterns are mixed, with both good and bad areas of life. This has already been suggested by the evidence of the associations between behaviours: Table 6.12 suggested that while there are some strong associations, others are relatively weak and some are negative. The 'best' pattern of behaviour – non-smoking, non-heavy drinker, good diet and high exercise – describes only about one fifth to a quarter of women under 60, and fewer of men or older women. The 'worst' – smokers and heavy drinkers with poor diet and low exercise – includes very few women, and only 7 per cent of men. Women have some likelihood of 'better' patterns because of less commonly being moderate/heavy drinkers or, to a lesser extent, smokers, and their somewhat better diet.

Figures 6.2 and 6.3 show the odds, calculated for this sample of the population, on moving from one category to another, that is, of being a non-smoker if male, or being a non- or light drinker if a non-smoker or smoker, of having a good diet if a smoker and drinker, and so on. Three figures are given, one for each age group.

As the correlations of Table 6.12 suggested, both male and female non-smokers were more likely to be non-drinkers, with the correlation less strong at younger ages. Male non-smokers in the middle years had an odds of almost 2:1 of being non-drinkers, but smokers an approximately even chance of drinking or not. Women were, of course, less likely to be smokers or

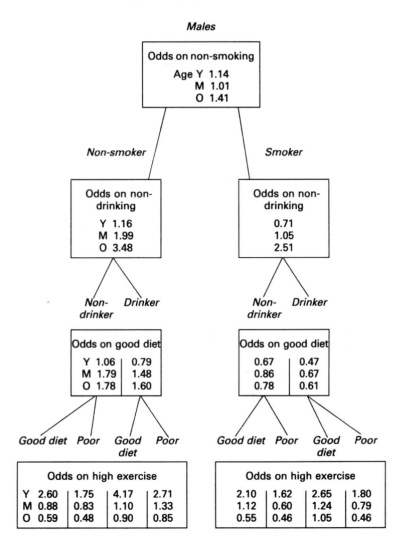

Figure 6.2 Odds on different combinations of behaviour, males

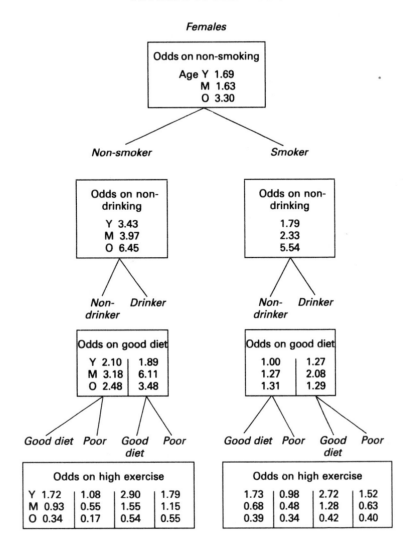

Figure 6.3 Odds on different combinations of behaviour, females

drinkers, but for young women non-smoking also doubled the odds on non-drinking.

Among men, the probability of a good diet was less for all smokers, but least for those who both smoked and drank. Among men over 60, for instance, odds on a good diet were only 0.6:1 for those who were smokers and drinkers, compared with 1.8:1 for those who were neither. Among women, the effect of the reverse correlations shown in Table 6.12 is evident. Women were, of course, quite likely to have a 'good' diet. Among non-smokers in the middle years, however, they were almost twice as likely to if they were drinkers. Smokers were much less likely to have good diets, but drinking smokers were more likely than non-drinking smokers. Only among young non-smokers, and more elderly smokers, were the odds on a good diet slightly greater if the individual was a non-drinker.

The odds on a high level of exercise obviously depended very much on age, ranging from over 4:1 among one behaviour group of young men, to only 0.17:1 among one group of older women. This regular relationship apart, however, some interesting patterns emerge at the last stages of Figures 6.2 and 6.3. Odds on high exercise were generally better for those whose diet was good. Among male smokers *and* non-smokers, however, drinkers had a higher probability of a high level of exercise than non-drinkers. Over 60, smokers and drinkers with a good diet were more than twice as likely to take vigorous exercise as non-smokers and non-drinkers with a poor diet. Among women, the association of high exercise with drinking, together with a good diet was even more marked, at younger ages. Smokers and non-smokers differed little, though in the middle years non-smokers had slightly higher probabilities of taking exercise, irrespective of drinking or diet.

It remains to be asked how patterns of behaviour are distributed in relation to characteristics other than age or gender – characteristics such as income, education, social class, area of residence, personal circumstances. The following descriptions are summaries of the most notable results of an analysis of the different patterns of behaviour shown in Figure 6.1 by these variables, considering particularly the more common combinations of behaviour. (Throughout, 'non-drinking' is used as a shorter description of 'not moderate/heavy drinker'.)

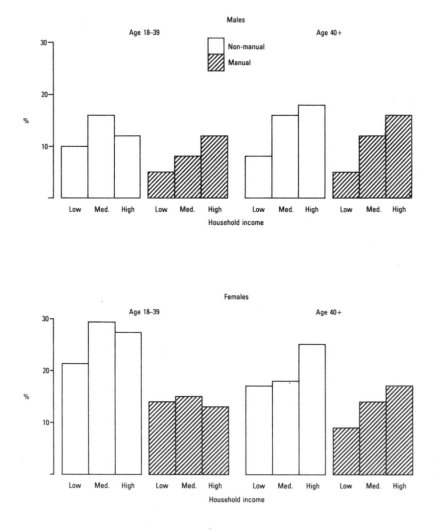

Figure 6.4 Income and behaviour: percentages of those with low, medium, or high household incomes who have 'completely healthy' behaviour, comparing non-manual and manual social classes

138

Behaviour all 'good': non-smoking, non-drinking, good diet and high exercise

Amongst men, irrespective of age, 10–11 per cent came into this behaviour category: there were more women, especially among the young, (21 per cent at 18–39 years). There was also a clear difference between non-manual and manual social classes, strongly related to education: totally 'good' behaviour patterns, at least as represented by these four areas of life, were most likely among people with better educational qualifications.

Income was also relevant. Irrespective of social class, those with low incomes were least likely to engage in this 'good' behaviour. Among older people, of whatever class, those with the highest incomes were most likely to be in this category. Interestingly, this was not necessarily true among younger men and women, however: the middle range of incomes, among non-manual men and women 18–39, was more favourable than the high (Figure 6.4). Younger people with the very highest incomes tended to fall short of the 'ideal' behaviour pattern, principally because of a greater likelihood of moderate/heavy drinking.

The occupations most likely to be represented in this 'good' behaviour pattern were those related to higher educational status: professional and technical or intermediate non-manual occupations. For instance, at ages 40–59, proportions of occupational groups with all 'good' behaviour may be compared: 32 per cent of male and 29 per cent of female professionals, or 29 per cent of male semi-professional or technical workers, and only 7 per cent or less of skilled or semi-skilled male workers. The group also included only 7 per cent of 'small' employers and managers at age 18–39. Unskilled workers, however, were not greatly under-represented. Among older people, employers and managers in large establishments – not small – were also well represented. Employed people were more likely to have this behaviour pattern than the unemployed, only 4 per cent of whom had totally 'good' behaviour. For men over 60, the typical representative of this category was retired rather than working. Overall, the income of the retired might be less, but comparing those with similar incomes, the retired individual was more likely to take exercise and also less likely to be a drinker.

Among women, on the other hand, the typical representative was working outside the home rather than a housewife – but working part-time rather than full-time. Younger men were more likely to have totally 'good' behaviour if married rather than single, especially if single and living alone or with companions of similar age. Younger unmarried women living in the parental home were particularly well represented (25 per cent of this group). At ages over 60 men – but not women – were better represented if they were living with a spouse, rather than widowed and living alone.

Regionally, totally 'good' behaviour was distributed in the ways which might be expected from the regional patterns of individual habits, with over-representation in the South East, South West and East Anglia, and under-representation in Scotland and all the northern regions. At small area level, the behaviour pattern was most common in 'high status' areas, and among non-manual people in cities and service centres.

Behaviour all 'good' except for one 'bad' habit

To have 'good' behaviour marred only by a lack of exercise was a common pattern among older men (18 per cent of those aged 60 and over) and women in the middle years and older (35 per cent of those aged 60 and over). Among young women, these were particularly likely to be junior non-manual workers, own-account workers or the wives of own-account workers. The wives of farmers and agricultural workers were prominent at all ages among women, as were men over 60 who had retired from agricultural occupations. This pattern of behaviour was also common among professional men and women, and the wives of professional men, in the middle and later years. It was another pattern of the married rather than the single, and among older men (but not women), the married rather than the widowed. Housewives, rather than employed women, tended to come into this category, rather than the category of 'ideal' behaviour which did include a high level of exercise. Among both men and women under 60, income was not strongly associated with the likelihood of this behaviour pattern, but among non-manual men and women over 60, those with low incomes were more likely to spoil their record of healthy behaviour by a lack of exercise.

Small proportions of men and women with otherwise good

habits were smokers. Non-manual social class and higher income within class were associated with this behaviour pattern, relatively common among employer/manager groups. This is a behavioural group whose health may be particularly interesting, since this one habit, undoubtedly unfavourable for health, occurs within a lifestyle which is otherwise favourable in both socio-economic and behavioural terms.

Moderate/heavy drinking, combined with no smoking, good diet and high exercise, is another behaviour pattern in which the effects of a single 'bad' habit can be examined in due course. This was strongly associated with higher income, and professional or managerial occupational classes predominated. For instance, 24 per cent of young men aged 18–39 in professional occupations had this behaviour pattern, compared with only 9 per cent of all men of this age. The typical representative of this group was single, if young, and living in London or the South East, or in 'high status' areas in other parts of the country.

Poor diet, as a single risk factor, was again more likely among men and among the young. Junior non-manual occupations were associated with this behaviour pattern, and also unskilled and own-account work among men and service occupations among women.

'Mixed' patterns of behaviour

As Figure 6.1 showed, many 'mixed' patterns of behaviour represent only small groups. Two patterns were prominent at particular ages, however: poor diet and low exercise combined with non-drinking and non-smoking among the elderly, and poor diet and drinking combined with non-smoking and a high level of exercise among the young.

Poor diet and low exercise combined with non-smoking and non-drinking was the pattern for 11 per cent of men over 60, and 16 per cent of women over 60, but smaller proportions of younger people. It was a lifestyle marked particularly by a likelihood of poverty, and most common amongst those whose occupations were, or had been, in service, semi-skilled and unskilled work. Amongst young women it was common among single-handed parents. Amongst the retired, it was most likely among older men living alone and older women living with their adult children or other relatives. Individuals with this behaviour pattern commonly lived in industrial, manufacturing, or rural areas. A high proportion of those below retirement age were wives not working outside the home, or their husbands, in families with children, in the North, Yorks and Humber and West Midland regions. This is a group whose health may be of particular interest: as non-smokers, they may be expected to have an advantage, but typically many other aspects of their lifestyle are unfavourable for health.

The common behaviour pattern among young men – non-smoking, and a high level of exercise, but accompanied by a poor diet and moderate/heavy drinking – may also be of interest in comparison with those who are similar but do smoke. This was a diverse group, consisting primarily of students, junior non-manual and clerical workers, and young skilled manual workers. This pattern was, again, typical of the North rather than the South.

Behaviour all 'bad': smoking, drinking, poor diet and low exercise

About 7 per cent of men, but few women, came into this category. Notably, they were the unemployed among the young (11 per cent of this group), married (but without children) or single but living alone, and among the elderly again those living alone. This 'consistently bad' behaviour pattern occurred at twice the average rate in the Northern and Yorks/Humber regions. Unskilled manual workers and their wives were the occupational group most likely to be represented, but there were also relatively high rates of 'all bad' behaviour among younger men in skilled jobs, employers/managers in 'small' establishments and their wives, foremen and supervisors among men of middle years, and those who had been in agricultural work among retired men.

Behaviour all 'bad' except for one good habit

Who were the people with generally 'unhealthy' behaviour who nevertheless had one area of life which might prove protective? Rather few individuals – 2–3 per cent overall – combined smoking, drinking, and low exercise with a good diet: the most common occupational class was that of 'small' employers/ managers. Similarly, few people combined heavy/moderate drinking, poor diet and low exercise with an absence of smoking (4 per cent of men and 2 per cent of women): these were most likely to be semi-skilled and service workers, predominantly in the northern regions.

Rather larger proportions, especially of young men (12 per cent) combined an otherwise unhealthy lifestyle with a high level of leisure exercise. These young men were likely to be in semi-skilled and unskilled occupations. They were more likely to be in this category if unemployed (17 per cent of the unemployed) and single rather than married.

Those who tempered an otherwise unhealthy lifestyle by abstention from moderate/heavy drinking, on the other hand, were more likely to be the elderly among men. Elderly women, of course, were more likely to be non-smokers as well. At all ages men and women who were married and with children were over-represented, compared with the single. Women working as housewives were more likely to be in this behaviour category than those employed outside the home, and unemployed men considerably more likely than the employed (for instance, at ages 40–59, 17 per cent of the unemployed and 7 per cent of the employed). This was a behaviour pattern most commonly found, especially for women, in Wales and Scotland. The occupational group which was prominent was that of semi-skilled and unskilled workers and their wives.

Income and unfavourable behaviour patterns

This description of the people with three, or four, 'unhealthy' behaviours suggests that general social class or income patterns are the reverse of those shown in Figure 6.4. As Figure 6.5 demonstrates, it is true that people with low incomes, and in manual rather than non-manual classes, were more likely to have at least three unhealthy areas of their lifestyle. However, it is only among mid-age men that class, and income within class, produce regular differences: those in non-manual jobs were always less likely to have generally unhealthy lives than those in manual jobs, and those with low incomes more likely than those with high. It can be noted that in fact a smaller proportion of manual men with high incomes led unhealthy lives, in terms of these four behaviours, than of non-manual men with low incomes. Among younger and older men, however, the class dimension seems dominant, with little effect of income. Among women, on the other hand, the effect of income appears to predominate over that of class.

Conclusion

It can always be shown, as it was in the earlier part of this chapter, that the major health-related behaviours are associated with social class, and education, and income, and regions of the country: those who are in the most disadvantaged circumstances are least likely to behave 'healthily'. This might support the view that the patterns of health typical of those in particular social situations, discussed in Chapter 5, are to some extent a consequence of, or at the least are reinforced by, voluntary ways of living.

There are several ways in which this is an over-simple view, however. One, which the later part of this chapter has been able to demonstrate, is that – even confining consideration to only these four areas of life – the majority of people do not have totally healthy or unhealthy lifestyles: most are mixed. This is true cross-sectionally, at the one moment of time represented by this survey. *Change* in behaviour is not documented, though the longitudinal, dynamic picture must be even more complex: in one national survey, 47 per cent of the respondents claimed that some change in their health-related behaviour had taken place in the previous ten years (Cartwright and Anderson 1981). It is *patterns* of behaviour, or the interaction of different habits, which will have to be examined in subsequent chapters, as possible determinants of health.

A second issue, which cannot be adequately dealt with in this analysis, is that patterns of behaviour have to be seen within the context of individual lives. 'Behaviour' has here been narrowly defined in terms of medically approved practices. However, many people may consider other behaviours more important. Alternatively, they may see these specific areas of life as important, but not for health reasons. Health benefits are often seen as only incidental reasons for adopting or giving up particular behaviours (Anderson 1983).

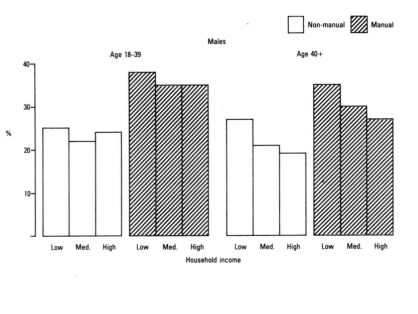

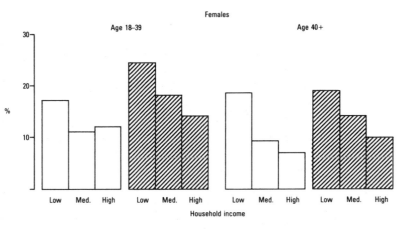

Figure 6.5 Income and behaviour: percentages of those with low, medium or high household incomes who have at least three 'unhealthy' behaviours, comparing non-manual and manual social classes

To select specific areas of life a priori is only one possible approach to 'health behaviour'. Another is to ask what people themselves define as health-promoting. It may well be that the activities which have been dealt with here, though they would be prominent on any health educator's list, are not necessarily related to health in the individual's mind. Moreover, these 'habits' may be just that: the four behaviours considered are very familiar everyday actions which may be automatic or taken-for-granted aspects of life. To what extent are patterns of behaviour dictated – for good or ill – by attitudes and beliefs, and what do people themselves count as health-related behaviour? These are the topics to be considered next.

Chapter Seven

ATTITUDES AND BEHAVIOUR

Obviously, behaviours affect health, though their relative importance, compared with other aspects of lifestyle, remains to be considered. It would also seem likely that attitudes are in some way related to the way in which people choose to live. Attitudes may be susceptible to change through health education: thus it is argued that 'the effectiveness of a preventive strategy depends to a large extent on people's attitudes and behaviour. This general thesis is well worth stating right from the start' (DHSS 1976: 6). The problematic area of this 'general thesis', however, lies in the relationship between attitudes and behaviour. This is a complex subject, on which there is a great body of research (for reviews see, e.g., Wallston and Wallston 1978, Anderson 1984, Dean 1984) and which cannot be dealt with in its entirety here. However, since the Health and Lifestyle Survey did include many questions about beliefs and attitudes, the opportunity does arise to explore some aspects of this relationship. In particular, what is the importance of attitudes, as intervening between social circumstances and the patterns of behaviour described in the previous chapter?

The concept of 'attitudes' is – like the concepts of 'health' or 'lifestyle' – a complex one. Some of the confusion in this field arises from a lack of clarity in what is meant by 'attitudes to health'; values, beliefs, intentions and general orientations may all be included.

Health is usually considered to be a very salient value. It is not necessarily true, however, that it is equally important for all groups of the population, nor are models of behaviour likely to be successful if they *assume* that health is valued above all other

147

aspects of life, or that health as a goal monopolizes human intentions. Health is often valued only in its absence: as Chapter 3 noted, many people said, 'You don't think about health until you're ill'. It is part of common experience that older people tend to give more importance to health than the young, and that those whose lives are very occupied may claim, while healthy, to 'have no time to think about their health'. In a national survey of the 'quality of life', only 10 per cent of the respondents included health as one of the dimensions affecting life quality, with more women than men, particularly in middle age, thinking that health was important (Hall 1983). The Health and Lifestyle Survey offered the statement 'to have good health is the most important thing in life' and respondents were asked to indicate their degree of agreement or disagreement. The majority agreed. A substantial minority disagreed or were equivocal, however – over 40 per cent of women, and about a third of men – and these were more likely to be the younger and better educated.

Health may be seen as a means to other valued ends, and not as an end in itself. It must not be presumed that 'healthy' behaviour is always purposive, and based on positive intentions to preserve health: young men, for instance, may find many quite different rewards in playing sports, or people may have moral rather than health-related attitudes towards heavy alcohol consumption. Similarly, if behaviour is 'unhealthy', and seemingly careless of the health consequences, it may be that it is simply not seen as relevant to health, or that the rewards outweigh any costs. Many behaviours regarded as undesirable by professionals may play an important part in individuals' coping strategies (Cameron and Jones 1985).

At this point the question arises of *beliefs*, defined as those things which people know or think to be true. Correct beliefs are a necessary preliminary to taking effective action, but beliefs do not necessarily predict either attitudes or behaviour. The great majority of the population, as will be shown later, believe that smoking is a cause of lung cancer. Holding this belief was only weakly associated with attitudes to smoking, however, and not at all with actually being a smoker or not.

Even given the existence of positive values and accurate beliefs, the barriers or facilitators which intervene between the intention to act 'healthily' and the action must be considered. It was noted in Chapter 6 that a 'healthy' diet is strongly class-related. To what extent is this explained by knowledge of the health implications of diet, or indeed attitudes to healthy living generally, and to what extent is it a function of income, the customs of the region in which one lives, or the everyday practicalities of life circumstances?

In spite of these problematic issues, it is clear that some interaction of values, beliefs, and perceptions of costs and benefits, modified by both external situations and by personality factors, must influence behaviour. Many models of these relationships have been developed by social psychologists. The best known is perhaps the Health Belief Model (Rosenstock 1969, 1974; Becker 1974) originally formulated to explain preventive health behaviour. Readiness to take a health action, it is suggested, is determined by the individual's perception of his own susceptibility and of the severity of the consequences of not taking the action, together forming the perceived threat. Given that this exists, the costs and benefits of taking the action are taken into account. Particular 'triggers' to action are also necessary, and personality factors or external circumstances may be modifying factors. Later developments of this model included a general concept of health motivation in order to improve its predictive power: a Health Action Model or Attitude-Behaviour Theory (Ajzen and Fishbein 1980) suggested that belief systems and general motivational systems acted multiplicatively, still with a necessity for 'enabling' factors to be present.

These models have had some success in studies of the take-up of screening services for particular diseases, but the results have not been consistent, and studies of more general health behaviour have shown them to be only weakly predictive (Harris and Guten 1979, Lindsey-Reid and Osborn 1980, Calnan 1984). As noted in Chapter 6, different types of 'health behaviour' must be distinguished: the factors which influence preventive behaviour (especially the use of preventive health services) and health-promoting lifestyles may be very different. Harris and Guten (1979), for instance, found that income and education were related positively with the use of preventive care, but negatively with other health practices.

As a general aid to understanding orientations to healthy

behaviour, a construct called 'health locus of control' has been much used (Wallston and Wallston 1978, Wallston *et al.* 1976). This may have more relevance to the survey described here, in which it is not possible to study *change* in behaviour. Behaviour which is positively directed at the goal of 'becoming healthy' requires reinforcement: the belief that this reinforcement is in one's own hands is described as an 'internal' locus of control. Belief in outside forces, such as chance or the actions of others, is referred to as 'external'. A high value given to the outcome, combined with an internal locus of control, is more likely to lead to behaviour such as reducing smoking (Kaplan and Cowles 1978). Single scales have not been found to be always successful in predicting actions, however, and this has led to multi-dimensional measures. For instance, externality has been separated into two components, belief in chance or fate and belief in control by powerful others (Levenson 1974; Wallston *et al.* 1978). Even these, however, have not always been able to predict people's awareness of the importance of behaviour in influencing their health (Pill and Stott 1981).

The general presumption behind these models is that if individuals are concerned about health, and believe that action can be taken which will be protective, then (if there are no insuperable barriers) change in behaviour will result. If beliefs about the consequences of actions are 'correct', then behaviour will be healthy. To what extent does this appear to be true in the Health and Lifestyle Survey?

Informtion on attitudes in the survey

The study included a great deal of information on beliefs, opinions and attitudes, not all of which can be dealt with here. The major questions that will be addressed in this chapter, however, include:

• Where do people perceive the springs of health and ill health to be located? What do they see as healthy and unhealthy in their own lives? Do they think of health as something outside the individual's control, or as something which is their own responsibility?

• Do they think about the causes of ill health differently in different contexts? Do they, for instance, apply knowledge in the abstract to their own experience? To what extent does their own health experience determine the way in which they think about the causes of ill health?

• To what extent do people claim to think about the health consequences of their own behaviour? What relationship do claims to behave healthily bear to the 'actual' behaviour which they describe? For whom is health a major life value? What relationship does this have to positive attitudes? Which carries the most weight in 'determining' choices of behaviour – attitudes or social circumstances?

The large-scale survey method has limitations in the attempt to answer these questions, as was noted in Chapter 3 in relation to general concepts of health. There is a great danger of receiving only 'approved' answers to simple, direct questions: if asked 'Is smoking good for you?' the great majority of respondents would doubtless reply 'no', This may mean no more than they know this to be the expected answer, and does not necessarily imply that they really believe it to be an important cause of ill health.

Various methods were employed in this survey in an attempt to minimize these problems. All the questions about beliefs and attitudes were asked early in the interview, before the answers could become 'contaminated' by the later, detailed, enquiry about specific behaviours. It is of course possible that people, remembering the opinion they had offered, then edited their accounts of their behaviour. There is no evidence that this happened, however, and all the experience of interview studies suggests that it presumes a better memory, and a greater strain towards rationality, than that which people normally exhibit in long conversations or interviews. All the questions about attitudes or beliefs were open-ended, with the respondents replying in their own words. It is suggested that these replies, offering what came first into people's minds or what seemed most important to them, are more meaningful than forced, pre-coded answers which put words into people's mouths. One problem of this method, however, is that multiple answers are always possible, and since, in general, younger and better educated respondents tended to offer a wider range of replies, they may automatically be represented in more different categories of answer. In order that this may be taken into account in interpreting tables in this chapter, the mean number of replies offered by each group is shown wherever it appears to be particularly relevant.

Some of the data to be presented relies on the answer to single questions. For the most part, however, the questions were designed to be analysed not as individual items of information but as part of indices which represent attitudes and beliefs expressed in many different contexts. The answers to single questions are not always meaningful: people are not inevitably consistent, nor should they be expected to be. However, if, when offered many different contexts in which it might be appropriate to reply 'I think that diet is very important here', an individual seizes every opportunity to do so, then that person can legitimately be characterized as one who thinks that diet is a salient issue for health. At a more general level, those who continually and throughout the interview stress the importance of self-responsibility and individual behaviour can be identified. The 'attitudes' used in Table 7.3 (sources of health/ill health), or Table 7.8 (importance of diet, etc.), are derived in this way.

These attempts at greater sophistication of analysis notwithstanding, it must always be borne in mind that the attitudes and opinions expressed in this, as in any relatively superficial survey, are 'presentations' to an interviewer: it cannot be pretended that we know what relationship they bear to what people 'really' think. Cornwell (1984), for instance, has identified substantial differences between 'public' accounts obtained at a first interview, giving what was thought to be acceptable answers, and 'private' accounts emerging only after several interviews. To map the prevailing acceptable public view is not without interest of itself, and the differences between social groups in the extent to which they are aware of that view or anxious to subscribe to it are also important. In associating opinions with behaviour, however, the problematic status of these attitudes must be taken into account.

The sources of health and ill health

Three sets of beliefs can be compared here: the causes of health and ill health, as general concepts, in society at large; the causes, specifically, of diseases; and the sources of health and ill health as the respondents perceived them in their own lives.

In all three contexts, individual behaviours were prominent. It seemed that the public had learned well the lessons of health education, and answers about 'healthy lifestyles' were the ones which came first to their minds, or ones which they saw as the 'correct' or expected replies. Emphasis differed, however, in the three different contexts.

The most general beliefs about the sources of health were elicited from the first two questions of the survey, asking respondents why they thought that people might be healthier, or less healthy, 'than in your parents' time' (Table 7.1). The intention here was not to test any knowledge of trends over time (the period referred to would, in any case, depend on the age of the speaker) but simply to see what areas of life, or categories of cause, came first to people's minds. Most respondents, very sensibly, offered some reasons why health in general was improving, and others which they thought caused a deterioration. It is perhaps of interest to note, however, that about one fifth of the sample insisted that they could think of no reasons why health might be better, or said 'it is not true that health is better nowadays'. This pessimistic view was most likely to be expressed by older people, especially women, and/or those with the lowest incomes, and/or those with the lowest educational qualifications. The opposite view – that there were no reasons why health might be worse nowadays – was extremely rare. In view of the general improvement in life expectancy, and the undoubted advances which medicine has achieved (mentioned, indeed, by many, as Table 7.1 shows), it seems a little difficult to explain why so large a proportion of the population believes that 'people are not healthier', particularly among the elderly who might have been expected to be exposed to the greatest change. At one level it appears that they are aware of the advances, but at another there would seem to be a strong perception of 'the unhealthiness of modern living', especially among older people: 'health' is not the same as life expectancy. Also, of course, there may be some element of the well-known phenomenon of seeing the past as always better than the present, exemplified in other areas by the belief that, for instance, society used to be less violent or more law-abiding. The common perception that

153

Table 7.1 Principal beliefs about the causes of health and ill health for society in general, comparing genders and age-groups

	Males			Females		
	Age 18–39	49–59	60+	18–39	40–59	60+
	Percentage of group					
Reasons volunteered why people are healthier nowadays						
Medical advances, medical care, changed patterns of disease, new drugs	42	35	34	38	30	24
Better diet, eating habits	33	37	31	45	44	30
Prosperity, standard of living	19	20	24	20	25	25
Health knowledge, education	23	13	6	25	16	9
Increased exercise	12	8	6	12	6	6
Working conditions, types of work	8	7	8	3	3	6
Hygiene, cleanliness	5	3	4	5	3	3
Public Health, environment	4	5	3	4	2	2
Decreased smoking, low tar cigarettes	3	2	2	2	2	1
Mean no. of reasons suggested	1.8	1.8	1.6	1.8	1.8	1.5
Reasons volunteered why people are less healthy nowadays						
Poorer diet, eating habits	23	22	19	28	31	26
Stress, pace of life	17	24	19	16	23	19
More smoking	14	14	17	16	16	15
Less exercise	15	14	14	12	12	11
Greater alcohol consumption	13	13	15	13	13	12
General behaviour	10	11	13	8	10	13
Environment, pollutants, etc.	10	8	7	9	8	5
Illegal drugs	6	6	8	6	5	6
Poverty, declining standard of living	6	7	5	6	6	6
Poorer working conditions	4	4	2	2	2	1
Unemployment	4	3	2	4	2	1
Changed patterns of disease	3	3	3	2	3	3
Deterioration in family/ community life	1	1	1	2	2	2
Mean no. of reasons suggested	1.4	1.5	1.5	1.4	1.4	1.5
(N = 100%)	(1,668)	(1,240)	(997)	(2,150)	(1,596)	(1,352)

smoking had *increased* since 'your parents' time' may be noted, and the relative prominence given to illegal drugs. Differences between men and women, and between age-groups, are also of interest. Younger people more frequently mentioned medical advances, education, and exercise; women placed more importance on food and diet and on standard of living, and men on medicine and on exercise.

To what extent are people's own circumstances associated with such general views about what influences health? The beliefs that health is better nowadays because of medical advances, or because of education and knowledge about health, were strongly associated with higher education and higher income: for instance, among men, 54 per cent of those with degree or professional-level education mentioned medicine and 30 per cent mentioned lay knowledge, compared with 30 per cent and 8 per cent respectively of those with no educational qualifications. The general category of psychological factors, notably the damaging effects of stress listed in Table 7.1, was also favoured by those with higher education, and particularly by men and women in the middle years of life rather than the young or the old. Conspicuously, it was cited by those who, in their answers to other questions, said that they were themselves 'under strain' – by 43 per cent of men aged 18–39 who said that they were often or always under strain, for instance, compared with only 11 per cent of those who said that they were never under strain.

Diet and exercise were behaviours that were mentioned more frequently by those in higher educational groups, though socio-economic characteristics did not appear to differentiate those who stressed alcohol and smoking. The respondents' own smoking or drinking habits did, however, show some association. As Table 7.2 shows, among younger people it was certainly not true that the 'guilty' smokers or drinkers were the ones who avoided mentioning these things as a cause of ill health. Over 60, however, smokers and female drinkers were less likely to volunteer general criticisms of these habits.

The causes of disease

Another set of questions in the survey asked the respondents what, in their opinion, caused eleven specific diseases. These

Table 7.2 Association of respondents' own smoking and drinking with the belief that the habits are reasons why people are less healthy nowadays

	Males			Females		
	Age 18–39	40–59	60+	18–39	40–59	60+
Smoking behaviour	*Percentage offering opinion that smoking causes ill health*					
Non-smokers	12	15	25	15	17	15
Ex-smokers	13	15	17	18	18	16
Smokers	16	15	11	18	16	10
Drinking behaviour	*Percentage offering opinion that drinking causes ill health*					
No alcohol	14	11	18	11	12	12
Light consumption	11	15	12	13	12	12
Moderate/heavy consumption	14	13	16	17	14	8
(N, smoking)	(607)	(231)	(131)	(991)	(666)	(696)
	(230)	(363)	(443)	(349)	(320)	(332)
	(780)	(618)	(414)	(799)	(606)	(314)
(N, drinking)	(375)	(392)	(403)	(978)	(785)	(912)
	(443)	(338)	(346)	(581)	(431)	(253)
	(849)	(510)	(248)	(591)	(380)	(187)

were chosen to represent the most common diseases which might be held to have some behavioural component, and excluded infectious diseases. The objective was not primarily to test accurate knowledge – for most of the conditions, cause may be held to be multiple and complex in any case – but, again, to see what areas of life were most prominent in people's minds as leading to ill health. For specific conditions, very varied answers were of course offered. Considering the whole range of replies, however, four major categories of cause emerged: personal behaviours (e.g. smoking, diet); the external environment (e.g. pollution, working conditions); heredity or inborn or acquired characteristics beyond the individual's control; and psycho-social factors, notably 'stress'.

Given the diseases chosen (e.g. lung cancer, 'a heart attack', chronic bronchitis, liver disease, high blood preassure) it is not surprising that 'unhealthy' behaviour was even more popular as a cause of specific disease. Lung cancer was said to be caused by ·smoking by 84 per cent of the respondents, and chronic bronchitis by 53 per cent. This may be compared with other surveys (e.g. Marsh 1985) where high proportions of the population agreed that smoking could be a cause of various diseases. In the Health and Lifestyle population, a majority associated heart disease with smoking, diet and overweight, or liver disease with an excess of alcohol. Younger men and women appeared to have accepted medicine's teaching about these diseases. Older people were more inclined to say that they did not know what the cause of a particular condition was, or to blame heredity or inborn susceptibility: notably, those who were themselves in poor health, or suffered from the specific disease being enquired about (and these were, of course, more likely to be elderly), were less ready to place the blame on behaviour. This seems very understandable: one may have bronchitis without, in fact, being a smoker, or even if a smoker, may be reluctant to admit self-responsibility for the disease. Many studies at a more intensive level have demonstrated that those who have a disease, or have close experience of it in others, are likely to develop elaborate and complex theories of causation (e.g. Blaxter 1983); this was tested in this survey by an examination of the ideas of cause held not only by those who suffered from a particular condition, but also those who said that a parent had died from it. It was confirmed that experience of a condition was certainly likely to make people think in terms of more complex, and less behavioural, causation. The fact that older people might be less likely to give simple 'approved' answers – 'heart disease is caused by a faulty diet' – must not, therefore, be seen simply as indicating less knowledge.

For those people without the disease in question, however, behaviour was associated with ideas of cause in the way that has already been illustrated: it was those *with* the relevant 'unhealthy' behaviour who were most conscious of the links with disease. For instance, 31 per cent of smokers said that smoking was one cause of 'a heart attack', compared with 20 per cent of non-smokers. Among those defined as obese, 35 per cent said that overweight was a cause of heart disease, compared with 21 per cent of those who were not themselves overweight. Among smokers, 62 per cent believed that smoking caused bronchitis, compared with 46 per cent of non-smokers. Drinkers were very much more aware of the association of alcohol and liver disease than non-drinkers. The only exception to this general rule was that, particularly among younger people, those who stressed the importance of diet in disease causation tended themselves to have 'healthy' diets.

It was noted in Table 7.1 that about a fifth of the respondents emphasized 'stress' or other psycho-social concepts when talking about the causes of ill health in general. A notable difference, when they were asked about the causes of diseases, was the additional weight given to this type of cause. Stress, worry, tension, unhappiness, disturbed family relationships, were offered as a cause for every type of condition. Over a quarter of the respondents said that these things caused heart attacks, for instance, and over half that they caused high blood pressure. Notably, this type of explanation was favoured more by those with higher education, and by those in the middle years rather than the young or the old. This emphasis on the psycho-social influences on health among men and women in their 40s and 50s is a trend which appears again and again in this survey.

Causes of disease associated with the physical environment were also more favoured by those with higher income or education, though here (with the exception of 'damp') more by younger people. In general, it begins to be obvious that a 'positive' attitude to health as something within one's own control, and a 'passive' attitude which implies that illness is imposed by outside forces, do not provide an easy dichotomy.

The sources of health and ill health in one's own life

Does the same apply, and are causes thought of in the same way, if people's minds are turned towards their own lives, rather than health and ill health in the abstract? They were asked whether there were any things about their lives at present which had a good effect, or a bad effect, upon their health; whether they thought they led a healthy life or not; and what their reasons were for thinking so. As with the questions about health in the abstract, most respondents gave both positive and negative replies. The answers to these questions are combined to form categories of 'beliefs about health in one's own life', providing categories of cause which are, of course, broadly similar to those which have been described. The education, knowledge, medical

Table 7.3 Comparison of the types of causes favoured, whether positively or negatively, in different contexts, comparing non-manual and manual social classes

Types of cause	For society at large				For one's own life				For a range of specific diseases			
	Male		Female		Male		Female		Male		Female	
	Non-man.	Man.	Non-man.	Man.	Non-man.	Man.	Non-man.	Man.	Non-man.	Man.	Non-man.	Man.
	Percentage of group stressing particular categories of cause											
Individual behaviour – diet, exercise, smoking, etc.	76	65	76	70	56	47	42	37	91	84	95	90
The external environment, incl. housing, pollution, etc.	22	26	23	25	19	17	21	15	39	39	33	24
Employment, unemployment, work generally	14	14	9	7	40	29	14	6	7	5	4	3
Standard of living, poverty or prosperity	30	26	31	26	8	5	6	7	negligible	negligible		
Family and social relationships	1	1	3	2	26	20	32	27				
Stress, contentment, psychological factors	29	16	25	16	33	21	38	30	78	74	82	76
Heredity and personal/family susceptibilities	negligible				4	2	5	5	18	10	20	9
(Mean no. of different categories mentioned by individuals)	(1.7)	(1.5)	(1.7)	(1.5)	(1.9)	(1.4)	(1.6)	(1.3)	(2.3)	(2.1)	(2.3)	(2.1)

(Multiple answers possible)

advances and medical care which had been prominent for improving the health of society at large are exceptions: only a handful of people mentioned any of these as having any relevance to the healthiness or otherwise of their own lives.

The emphasis on particular categories of cause changed, however, when the respondents were speaking of themelves. Comparisons between the three contexts – the health of society in general, the causes of disease, and one's own health – are shown in Table 7.3. Personal behaviours remained the most popular reason for suggesting that one's own life was healthy or unhealthy, but to a rather lesser degree than when thinking about 'other people', or society in general, as might be expected. Taking exercise was the behaviour most frequently offered as 'healthy' by men, especially the young, and exercise and diet were commonly cited by women, again especially the young. Smoking and/or lack of exercise were emphasized by men as 'unhealthy' factors in their lives, especially the middle-aged, and poor diets, overweight, and/or lack of exercise by women.

It can be noted in Table 7.3 that standards of living, general or personal prosperity or poverty, were quite commonly offered as influences on health in the general context, but rarely mentioned, for good or ill, as important for health in one's own life. When the incomes of those giving this type of reply were examined, it was notable that – whether talking about poverty or prosperity – they were more likely to be those in *more* favourable circumstances. Among those in a high family income group (£996+/month) 26 per cent thought that improving standards of living meant that people were, in general, healthier nowadays, and 9 per cent mentioned this as a good factor in their own lives. Among those in a low income group (<£416/month) the proportions were, as might be expected, lower: 19 per cent and 2 per cent. Fewer people mentioned the converse, poverty as a cause of ill health, but those with high incomes were twice as likely to do so in the general context as those with low incomes. Only 2–3 per cent focused on socio-economic factors in their own life, with little difference by income. The old – more likely to have low incomes – were particularly unlikely to mention the effects of poverty.

Similarly, housing tenure or social class made little difference to the likelihood of an emphasis on housing. Those living in cities (notably London) were more conscious of the effect of the general environment for ill health, and those in rural areas more likely to see their environment as good. However, as already noted, it was those in non-manual social classes, irrespective of area, who more readily talked about environmental factors.

Considering the area 'families' used before, it appeared that type of area of residence made little difference to thinking in terms of the environment when considering effects on health trends generally. Men and women in non-manual families remained more likely to mention environmental factors, for good or ill, whether they lived in rural areas or industrial areas. Certain differences did emerge when particular age-groups were considered: men (but not women) over 60 in rural areas and resort areas, *and* in cities, were especially conscious of the ill effects of pollution or city life. Older men, and women, in industrial areas, however, rarely mentioned these things.

There was, as might be expected, a greater effect of living area on consciousness of the environment as a factor in one's own life. Some of those in 'high status' areas mentioned it as favourable (18 per cent of men and 16 per cent of women, with particularly few under 40), and some in industrial or manufacturing areas saw the environment as detrimental (17 per cent of men and 15 per cent of women). Those in cities and 'high local authority housing' areas were less likely to cite their environment as important (in cities, 11 per cent of men and 14 per cent of women). The highest rates of declaring that their environment was a healthy factor in their own lives occurred in rural areas, wherever they were situated geographically (28 per cent of men and 23 per cent of women, with particularly high rates among elderly women) and resort/retirement areas (21 per cent of men and 22 per cent of women).

Respondents were considerably more likely to mention work (or the lack of it) or working conditions as a source of health or ill health when they were thinking of their own lives, but again it was a topic more frequently mentioned by those whose work might be presumed to be *less* harmful to health. Among men, two types of occupation were seen as particular sources of good health: agricultural occupations, and own-account small tradesmen. For the rest, however, semi- and unskilled workers were more likely to say that work was a healthy factor in their lives than were professionals, managers, or other non-manual workers. Professionals and employers/managers were in fact the groups most likely to feel that their work *harmed* their health, usually on the grounds of stress. Rather few women placed any emphasis on work, but again almost 10 per cent of those who themselves worked in clerical or other junior non-manual jobs believed that their work harmed their health, compared with very few who were themselves in manual jobs.

On the other hand, women were rather more likely than men to locate influences on health in family structures, social relationships and psychological factors, especially women in their middle years.

Summary: beliefs about causes

The major conclusions which may be drawn from this analysis of the beliefs about health which were presented include, firstly, that there is a high level of agreement within the population that health is, to a considerable extent, dependent on behaviour and in one's own hands. A survey cannot judge how deeply or sincerely these beliefs are held, but at the least it is recognized that these are the 'correct' or 'expected' answers to give. Beliefs about health as a general concept, and about disease, must be distinguished, as must beliefs about the health of society at large and about health in one's own life. In all these contexts, however, higher educational or social class groups, and the young, are more likely to emphasize 'voluntary' behaviours, but they are also more likely to emphasize some of the factors outside the individual's control. Those who, as Chapter 5 showed, are most prone to ill health – those in the poorest circumstances or environments – very rarely attribute their ill health to their situation; they, too, have learned to blame their own behaviour. Despite all the discussion at academic and political levels of 'inequalities in health', it seems that the issues are not seen as relevant at the level of individuals' own lives. Similar evidence has been offered by Calnan (1987) in a study comparing the views of women in social classes I/II and IV/V. Asked to compare the health of office workers and manual workers, a high proportion of the middle-class women believed the health problems to be equal, though different, and a majority of the working-class women said that office workers would have poorer health because of, for instance, inactivity. Similarly, in comparing the rich with the poor, the employed with the unemployed, or professionals with unskilled workers, those middle-class women who agreed that the less advantaged would have poorer health ascribed the cause primarily to psychological factors, and many of the working-class women said that these situations made no difference to health. As one explained:

> No, I shouldn't think it makes any difference myself. I mean ... people with money, they get the same illnesses as we get.
> (Calnan 1987: 79)

It remains to be asked, of course, what relationship these attitudes have to the deliberate intention to adopt 'healthy' behaviours, or indeed to the actual behaviours themselves.

THE 'HEALTHY' LIFE

When asked whether they thought they led a healthy life, most people replied 'quite healthy' or 'fairly healthy'. Substantial minorities however, said that their lifestyle was 'very healthy', or that they led unhealthy lives. About 20 per cent of males, and a slightly smaller proportion of females, believed that they led a 'very healthy life'. At the other extreme, about 10 per cent of both genders said that their lifestyle was 'unhealthy'. The likelihood of thinking one's life healthy increased very regularly with age, with, for instance, 15 per cent of men under 40 claiming a healthy life, compared with 29 per cent over 60. There was no regular trend by social class, nor were work or its nature clearly associated with believing one's lifestyle to be healthy, except that the unemployed over 40 were particularly likely to think their life unhealthy. Among women, working outside the home, rather than as a housewife, was significantly associated with a more positive view of lifestyle.

The characteristics which most clearly distinguished the optimistic and the pessimistic, however, were the three illustrated in Table 7.4. Living in a rural area was strongly associated with thinking one's lifestyle healthy, especially for women. Again especially for women, there was also a strong association with the measure of 'perceived social support': those who felt themselves to be isolated or without close emotional support from others were the most likely to think their lives unhealthy. The objective measure of social integration, distinguishing those with many activities and relationships and those with few, was less important, but those with many activities were unlikely to call their lives unhealthy.

Table 7.4 Characteristics associated with thinking that one leads a healthy life

	Percentage saying that their own life is:								
	Very healthy	Not healthy	(N)	Very healthy	Not healthy	(N)	Very healthy	Not healthy	(N)
	Age 18–39			40–59			60+		
Perceived social support									
Males									
No lack of support	18	9	(900)	22	9	(710)	33	6	(620)
Severe lack of support	11	18	(215)	16	11	(144)	16	11	(125)
Females									
No lack of support	15	5	(1,345)	19	6	(1,025)	25	6	(896)
Severe lack of support	7	18	(180)	9	20	(128)	15	16	(170)
Social Integration									
Males									
High	15	9	(633)	20	6	(511)	28	3	(65)
Low	16	14	(287)	18	16	(192)	28	8	(431)
Females									
High	13	5	(578)	20	5	(384)	—	—	
Low	12	14	(418)	15	13	(381)	23	9	(875)
Area of residence									
Males									
Rural	18	6	(278)	26	8	(251)	33	6	(214)
City	15	12	(621)	21	10	(384)	26	5	(330)
Females									
Rural	15	5	(389)	21	8	(358)	32	4	(260)
City	10	9	(774)	14	11	(485)	19	11	(460)

Healthy and unhealthy behaviour

A high proportion of those who said that they led a healthy, or an unhealthy, life gave a reason associated with their own behaviour. All respondents were also asked whether they did anything 'to keep yourself healthy or improve your health' and whether there were 'things you would like to do to keep yourself healthy but don't do'. This is a self-defined approach to the definition of healthy behaviour which allows for the identification of other things than the conventional risk factors. In fact, although the questions were asked before the detailed enquiries about diet, exercise, smoking and alcohol consumption, which might have alerted or reminded the respondents, these four behaviours – especially exercise – were very prominent.

Figure 7.1 shows that claiming to take active steps towards health did not differ greatly between age-groups: the elderly, though they might cite different activities, could still mention health-promoting activities. Social class differences, growing less with age, were marked.

Though these proportions of people claiming to 'do things' to promote their health are high, it can be noted that they are considerably less than the 97 per cent reported in the United States survey in which the same questions were asked (Harris and Guten 1979). In that survey, answers about diet were conspicuously the most popular, offered by 70 per cent. Here, diet was also a favoured answer, though more among non-manual than manual social classes, and among women than men (Table 7.5). Exercise was, however, by far the most popular answer here, both as an activity undertaken and as the thing which people wished they did more of. This was expressed as sports, or jogging and other keep-fit activities, among younger people and activity such as walking or gardening among the elderly. It can be noted that there was no social class difference among those claiming general activity, but a difference, especially among women, in taking part in active sports or keep-fit. No other 'healthy behaviours' were claimed or aspired to by more than small proportions, nor were there other differences by social class except that men in manual work were more likely than those in non-manual jobs to say that their work kept them healthy. The 6 per cent of men and 5 per cent of women who wished to stop smoking were evenly distributed by social class.

Health and claims to 'do things to keep healthy'

Considering the summary categories of health status (p. 54), there were considerable differences both in claiming to do

165

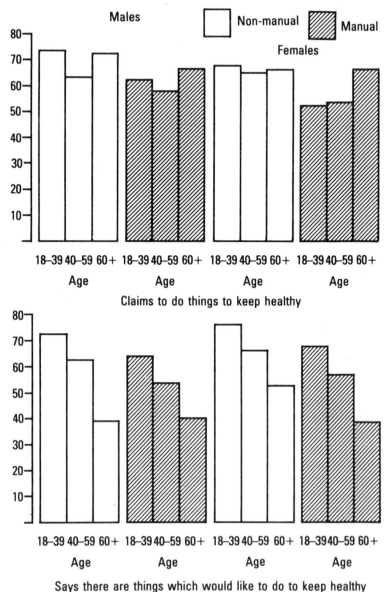

Figure 7.1 Percentages of men and women who say that they do 'things to keep healthy', or that they would like to do (other) things, comparing non-manual and manual social classes

Table 7.5 Types of behaviour volunteered as things done 'to keep healthy' or things the respondent 'would like to do', comparing ages and social classes

	Males					Females				
	Age 18–39	40–59	60+	NM	M	18–39	40–59	60+	NM	M
Things claimed to be done to keep healthy	*Percentage of group*									
Active sports, keep fit	61	24	20	35	28	43	25	14	34	21
Other activity (e.g. gardening, walking, 'take exercise')	15	30	58	25	26	19	28	41	24	23
Diet	14	13	13	19	9	24	23	20	29	18
Watch/reduce weight	2	3	2	3	2	7	7	3	6	6
No/moderate smoking	4	5	5	3	3	3	3	2	3	2
No/moderate alcohol	2	2	2	3	2	1	1	1	2	1
Social activities	1	1	4	2	2	1	2	5	2	2
Mental attitudes	2	2	3	3	2	1	2	3	2	2
Medical treatment	1	1	4	2	2	2	3	6	3	3
Work keeps healthy	10	13	8	7	13	3	6	3	4	4
Environment keeps healthy	3	3	8	4	5	3	5	7	4	4
Other and vague (e.g. 'moderation')	3	4	10	6	5	3	8	10	8	5
(mean no. of things done)	(1.2)	(1.0)	(1.4)	(1.2)	(1.1)	(1.1)	(1.1)	(1.2)	(1.2)	(1.0)
Things would like to do to keep healthy										
More exercise	54	41	24	47	39	59	42	25	50	40
Alter diet	5	3	1	6	2	8	6	2	7	5
Lose weight	2	2	1	3	1	5	6	3	5	5
Stop/reduce smoking	7	7	4	6	6	6	6	2	5	5
Stop/reduce alcohol	2	1	0	1	1	0	1	0	1	1
Change social activities	2	2	5	3	2	1	3	4	3	2
Change/get job	1	3	2	2	2	0	1	2	1	2
Other and vague (e.g. 'lead a healthier life')	4	3	6	4	4	3	4	4	3	4
(mean no. of things would like to do)	(0.8)	(0.6)	(0.4)	(0.7)	(0.5)	(0.8)	(0.7)	(0.4)	(0.8)	(0.6)

'things to keep healthy' and in being ready to say that there were things 'you would like to do but do not'. The relationship between health and actual behaviour is a topic for Chapter 8: the question here is the extent to which states of health affect the likelihood of *claiming* health-promoting activities.

The lowest rates of claiming to perform health-protective actions were found among those in the 'high illness without disease' and 'good physical health but poor psycho-social health' categories, especially in the middle years. Only 51 per cent of women, and 52 per cent of men, aged 40–59 years, in the poor psycho-social health category presented a positive attitude to health promotion, for instance. Those who were in the 'good health but unfit' group, among women under 60 but not men, were similarly less likely to claim active health behaviour.

Two groups were particularly likely to say that they took active steps to promote health: the above-average healthy, and those in the worst health. Men, especially, in excellent overall health said this: for instance, 85 per cent of those over 60. Among those with chronic conditions, whether or not they were 'limiting', about 70 per cent of men and 65 per cent of women in all age-groups claimed health-promoting behaviour.

'Wanting to do things to keep healthy' – i.e. being conscious that behavioural habits were relevant, but not claiming to adopt them – was, as has been shown, less common among the elderly than the young, and this was true whatever the health status group. Here, too, those who were in good health but were unfit were unlikely to be prominent. Men and women in the good or excellent health categories, especially if older, were also less likely to be able to think of actions they should take, but did not. Those of all ages who were in the 'poor psycho-social health only' and 'illness without disease' categories, however, demonstrated that their inability to mention health-promoting behaviours that they performed was not a general carelessness or belief that behaviour was irrelevant: they were particularly likely (especially among the young) to express guilt by mentioning things that they knew they ought to do. Men and women of all ages with very poor health were the most likely of all to say that there were health-promoting things they would like to do, but did not (for instance, 60 per cent of women over 60 in the 'worst' health category, and 85 per cent of women aged 18–49).

Reported behaviour and 'actual' behaviour

On the whole, those who claimed to carry out specific 'healthy' actions were found to perform them, when asked in detail about the relevant area of life. There were only very small proportions whose claims appeared to be contradicted by their actions.

Those who said that their abstinence or moderate drinking was a health-promoting behaviour drank much less, on average, than those who said they ought to drink less. Those who claimed not smoking, giving up smoking, or reducing their smoking were likely to be non-smokers, or at least to smoke less than those who said that smoking was a behaviour they would like to change; those who said that their weight was too heavy, more likely to be overweight or obese. Some examples are shown in Tables 7.6 and 7.7. As might be expected, however, groups demonstrated different norms about what constituted, for instance, the 'right' weight, or 'enough' exercise, or 'moderate' drinking. It has also to be noted that high proportions of those whose behaviour *was* healthy did not think to mention it specifically as something which they did to keep or promote their health.

Table 7.6   Mean weights of those who do, or do not, say that they would like to lose weight

	Males		Females	
	Age 18–39	40–59	18–39	40–59
	Mean (measured) weight, kg.			
Wants to lose weight				
Yes	89.3	87.8	72.8	75.3
No	73.4	77.1	60.3	64.1

At a more general level, the earlier questions about 'Do you lead a healthy or unhealthy life? What makes you say this?' and 'Are there things about your life that have a good/bad effect on your health?' may perhaps be more interesting to compare with 'actual' behaviour. These invite the respondent to consider behaviour in the context of other areas of life. As already noted, high proportions *did* mention diet and exercise, though fewer at this point thought of smoking or alcohol consumption. Figure 7.2 demonstrates the relationship between thinking that one's life was healthy because of exercise, diet, or smoking habits, and actual behaviour as defined by the behavioural indices of Chapter 6. (Alcohol consumption is omitted because relatively

Table 7.7　Percentage of non-smokers and smokers who claim that stopping or reducing smoking is a health behaviour which they have done or would like to do

	Age 18–39			40–59			60+		
	Non-smoker	<20/ day	20+/ day	Non-smoker	<20/ day	20+/ day	Non-smoker	<20/ day	20+/ day
Males									
Claims to have stopped/reduced	5	2	–	7	3	–	5	1	–
Would like to	–	17	30	–	18	18	–	11	19
(N=100%)	(1,043)	(525)	(100)	(787)	(323)	(130)	(727)	(228)	(42)
Females									
Claims to have stopped/reduced	4	1	1	4	1	2	2	2	–
Would like to	–	17	24	–	14	22	–	8	(4)
(N=100%)	(3,412)	(659)	(79)	(1,032)	(487)	(77)	(1,060)	(276)	(16)

few people mentioned it spontaneously, and those who did *not* mention it as a healthy factor in their lives were as likely to have no or light consumption as those who did. It seems that alcohol consumption is not readily thought of as a health behaviour, except by the small minority who are conscious that their drinking is too heavy, or are willing to admit this.)

Age-groups under and over 50 years are distinguished because of the difference in behaviour patterns (particularly exercise) between the younger and the older. It can be noted that those who claimed a healthy life because of more exercise, better diet, or no smoking, were indeed more likely to have 'better' habits than those who did not. Two thirds of the younger men who claimed that their life was healthy because of the exercise they took were categorized in the 'high' level of exercise, and three-quarters of those who emphasized smoking in their own lives were non-smokers. For each type of behaviour, people who had not claimed it were significantly more likely to be in the 'bad' categories. However, it is also obvious that there were quite substantial proportions of people who said that 'my life is healthy because I take exercise, or have a good diet, or smoke little or not at all,' who in fact appeared in the 'worst'

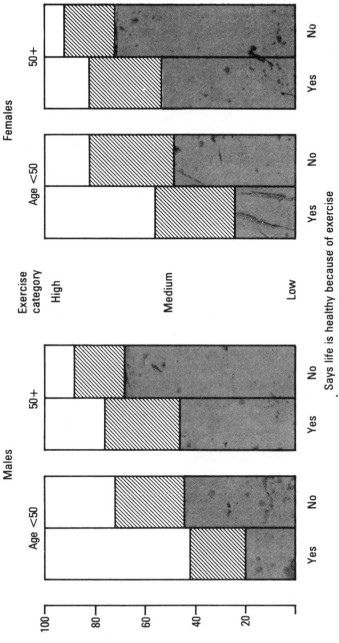

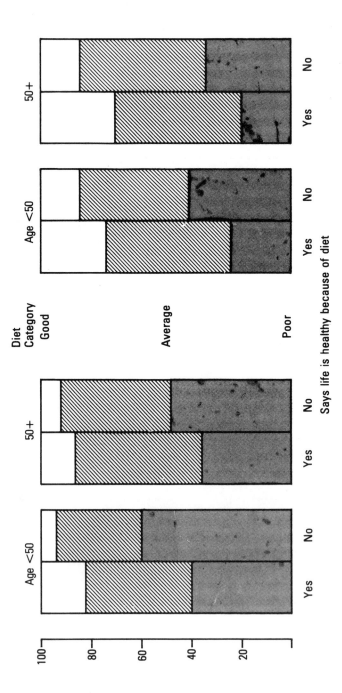

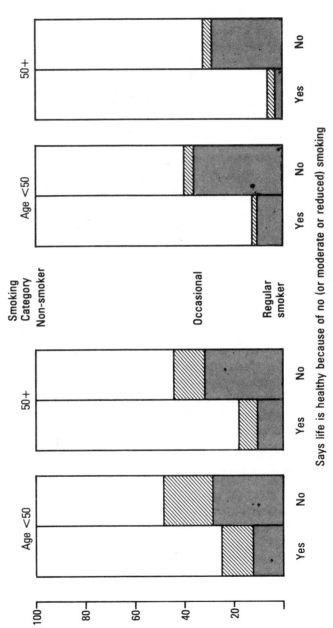

Figure 7.2 Percentage of those who say, or do not say, that their own life is healthy because of specific behaviours, whose 'actual' behaviour is 'healthy' or 'unhealthy'

categories when their lifestyles were examined in detail. This is particularly true of exercise among men and women over 50, and of diet among men. Since 'low' exercise, it will be remembered, is defined as at best only a very modest amount of e.g. walking or gardening, and certainly no vigorous exercise or sporting activities, during 'the past fortnight', it would seem that the claim to 'take exercise' can refer to only occasional activity.

Another notable point demonstrated in the diagram is that many people do have good diets, or exercise habits, or are non-smokers, without thinking of mentioning these things when asked why their lives are healthy. A third of the younger men who did not list exercise did in fact have high levels of sporting and other active leisure pursuits, and half of those who did not mention smoking were non-smokers. These patterns of behaviour are not necessarily motivated by health considerations. Alternatively, it is possible that lifestyles originally adopted with health seen as at least partly relevant – e.g. the decision not to smoke – may become routine and 'normal', and do not continue to be seen as active health practices. For whatever reason, it is clear that replies to survey questions which ask 'what do you do to keep healthy' are best interpreted as demonstrating *attitudes* to health, and must be treated with great caution as indicators of actual behaviour. People do not, on the whole, appear to attempt to deceive, but there are high proportions of 'false negatives'.

Belief that life is 'healthy' and overall behaviour patterns

So far, individual aspects of lifestyle have been considered. What of different combinations of the four behaviours? Considering the sixteen possible categories listed in Figure 6.1, it was clear that 'a healthy life' was being defined in terms of generally healthy *behaviour*. For both men and women, and for all age groups, the people most likely to say that they led a very *healthy* life were non-smokers with high exercise, though they might have a poor diet and be moderate/heavy drinkers. Only among some mid-age men and women was a 'very healthy' life perceived which did not include a high level of exercise. Some men and women over 60 were the only group of smokers to define their own lives as healthy, and then only if their exercise was high.

This suggests that *smoking* is the most salient factor of self-perceived healthy or unhealthy lifestyles. *Exercise* is also important: most of those with a low level of exercise defined their lives as unhealthy, even if other elements might be favourable. Moderate/heavy *drinking* or poor *diet* were less important, only being defined as an unhealthy lifestyle when combined with other 'bad' habits.

Relative importance of the four health behaviours

In addition to the questions, and indices derived from them, which were intended to 'measure' the respondents' attitudes to voluntary behaviour in general as a cause of health or ill health, measures of specific attitudes to each of the four health behaviours as health issues were derived. Indices called 'attitudes to smoking/diet/exercise/alcohol' were derived from the voluntary answers to a great many questions: the causes of health/ill health for society at large, and in the respondent's own life; what he or she does or would like to do as health-relevant behaviour; the causes of the range of specific diseases enquired about; and why (if they did) the respondents thought that ill health was 'people's own fault'. There were thus many occasions in the interview where an individual could mention, for instance, diet or smoking if they chose to. Some might mention smoking only once or twice: a very high proportion gave this answer when asked for the cause of lung cancer. Others might repeat their belief that smoking was an important factor for health generally, and as the cause of different diseases, many times throughout the interview. It is suggested that this method – more akin to the forms of analysis used in qualitative or more intensive research, and treating the interview as a whole – offers a better measure of how important issues actually are to the respondent.

Scales were formed for each 'attitude' and categories derived which indicate that the respondent gave 'high', 'average' or 'low' importance to each area of life in the context of health, which can be used comparatively (Appendix D). The proportions of people in different behavioural groups who gave a 'high' salience to each of the health-related habits is shown in Table 7.8. Fewer gave high importance to alcohol consumption than to the other behaviours: the areas of life most frequently mentioned were, as found before, diet by women and exercise by young men. Older men and women tended to have lower scores on all the indices, largely because (as noted earlier) they were less likely to ascribe either their own health status, or the causes of disease generally, to behavioural habits.

Table 7.8   Importance given to smoking, alcohol, diet or exercise as a health behaviour, by those with different behaviours (per cent)

Smoking: Importance given to smoking as a health behaviour	*Age* *18–39*		*40–59*		*60+*	
	Smokers	*Non-smokers*	Smokers	*Non-smokers*	Smokers	*Non-smokers*
Males						
High	45	35	39	34	21	29
Medium	36	38	29	37	38	37
Low	19	27	32	29	41	34
(N=100%)	(625)	(1,043)	(453)	(786)	(270)	(727)
Females						
High	42	34	33	34	17	19
Medium	37	38	39	39	35	34
Low	21	28	28	27	48	47
(N=100%)	(738)	(1,411)	(564)	(1,391)	(292)	(1,058)

Alcohol: Importance given to alcohol consumption as a health behaviour	*Age* *18–39*			*40–59*			*60+*		
	Mod/heavy drinkers	Light	*Non-drinkers*	Mod/heavy drinkers	Light	*Non-drinkers*	Mod/heavy drinkers	Light	*Non-drinkers*
Males									
High	21	12	17	18	15	15	16	11	16
Medium	34	32	29	34	28	26	34	35	29
Low	45	56	54	48	57	59	50	54	55
(N=100%)	(868)	(583)	(212)	(510)	(474)	(256)	(248)	(435)	(314)
Females									
High	13	10	10	11	11	8	5	7	6
Medium	31	25	28	29	27	25	27	22	22
Low	56	65	62	60	63	67	68	71	72
(N=100%)	(591)	(937)	(622)	(381)	(618)	(597)	(187)	(377)	(788)

Diet: Importance given to diet as a health behaviour		Age 18–39		40–59		60+	
		Poor diet	Good	Poor diet	Good	Poor diet	Good
	Males						
	High	26	53	23	45	18	35
	Medium	40	31	46	34	45	41
	Low	34	16	31	21	37	24
(N=100%)		(966)	(702)	(583)	(657)	(452)	(545)
	Females						
	High	38	74	32	70	17	46
	Medium	38	21	43	24	49	40
	Low	24	5	25	6	34	15
(N=100%)		(825)	(1,325)	(463)	(1,143)	(426)	(926)

Exercise: Importance given to exercise as a health behaviour		Low exercise	High	Low exercise	High	Low exercise	High
	Males						
	High	31	54	23	41	24	38
	Medium	47	40	49	44	48	46
	Low	21	6	28	15	28	16
(N=100%)		(516)	(1,152)	(648)	(592)	(631)	(336)
	Females						
	High	24	42	15	35	13	31
	Medium	52	49	48	49	45	49
	Low	23	10	37	17	41	20
(N=100%)		(828)	(1,322)	(871)	(725)	(1,017)	(335)

High scores on each of these scales were strongly associated with better education. This was particularly true for older people, for all four behaviours, and for diet and exercise, but not smoking or alcohol, among those under 60. Thus there were some marked social class and occupational differences: for example, 25 per cent of young women in unskilled families giving high importance to exercise, compared with 45 per cent in professional families, or 30 per cent of men in the middle years in skilled manual work giving high importance to diet compared with 49 per cent in employer/manager occupations.

For smoking, there were relatively small differences (under the age of 60) between non-manual and manual groups: agreement that this habit was relevant to health was more evenly distributed. For alcohol, there were negligible differences by education or social class: indeed, among women aged 40–59, those in manual families appeared to be more conscious of the link between excessive consumption and health.

When these attitude categories are related to actual reported behaviour, the results are consistent with those previously noted (e.g. Table 7.2). Smokers and moderate/heavy drinkers were more likely, among the young, to have emphasized the importance of these habits as health risks throughout the interview. At the same time, relatively high proportions of non-smokers or non-drinkers did not score highly on the 'salience' scales.

Exercise and diet are different, however. Small proportions of those whose lifestyles were 'healthy' in these respects failed to mention their importance in many different contexts: only 5 per cent of young women with good diets, for instance, had low scores on the 'salience of diet' scale and only 6 per cent of young men with high exercise had low scores on the 'salience of exercise' scale. At all ages, those with poor exercise or diet habits were less likely to express awareness of the health hazards. At this level, where characteristics such as education or income are not controlled for, there is a clear apparent association between attitudes to diet and exercise and actual behaviour.

HEALTH AS A VALUE AND HEALTH BEHAVIOUR

The above analyses have related to *beliefs* about health, and to attitudes defined narrowly as 'attitudes to specific healthy behaviours'. As noted at the beginning of this chapter, health attitudes may also be defined more generally, as a value or orientation towards a positive feeling of control over health. This survey cannot hope to match the sophistication of the wealth of psychometric research on these topics. There is, however, a variety of simple measures available (Appendix D): scores on a health locus of control instrument, degrees of agreement with the statement 'to have good health is the most important thing in life', and answers to the question 'Do you think it is people's own fault if they get ill?' The distributions of these are shown in Table 7.9.

178

Table 7.9 Distribution of attitudes to health

Percentage of gender/ age/class group who:	Age 18–39		40–59		60+	
	Non-man.	Man.	Non-man.	Man.	Non-man.	Man.
Males						
Have 'internal' locus of control	62	53	57	45	49	42
Believe ill health can be own fault	77	62	74	60	64	55
Believe health the most important thing in life	33	39	38	48	56	58
(N=100%)	(673)	(953)	(516)	(724)	(362)	(630)
Females						
Have 'internal' locus of control	54	47	46	42	39	35
Believe ill health can be own fault	68	60	65	54	55	51
Believe health the most important thing in life	42	43	52	57	64	62
(N=100%)	(994)	(1,119)	(727)	(852)	(515)	(806)

'Internal' locus of control and expresing the belief that illness is 'people's own fault' were associated, as might be expected, and more common among younger people, the better educated and those with higher incomes and/or non-manual social class. Age made less difference to the answers to the simple question about responsibility for health, however, than to the locus of control score. About two-thirds of all men and women agreed that people were 'guilty' of their own ill health, offering conventional reasons why this was so: smoking, unwise diet, lack of exercise, illegal drugs, general 'excess' or unhealthy lifestyles. The respondents' own state of health was, again, relevant, with those who were themselves in poor health less likely to take the 'self-responsible' view.

Health as a value was also associated positively with 'internal' locus of control. However – to the extent that such a complex concept can be 'measured' by one direct question – giving the highest value to health as the 'most important thing in life' was also associated with *lower* education and income, and was *more* likely among the old than the young. This is, of course, a common observation: health becomes a more pressing concern as one ages. Actual health status, relative to age, had rather little effect – more, in the middle years or among younger women. Young men in manual classes were more likely to give health the highest value if in fact their health was good, but in non-manual classes if it was in fact poor. The reverse relationship appeared to be true for older men and women: those in non-manual classes expressed a greater valuation of health if they were particularly healthy, and those in manual classes a greater valuation if they were suffering from chronic diseases.

Examined against 'actual' behaviour categories, it became clear that different behaviours have to be distinguished: these overall indicators of attitude are not related to all health-relevant actions in the same way. Those who thought that people were responsible for their own health, or were categorized as having 'internal' locus of control, were more likely to have good diets, and for most age-gender groups more likely to have high levels of leisure exercise. Within social classes, this was more evident among non-manual men and women. Among young men, however, there was little relationship with actual exercise. Association with smoking was less clear, for men, with little difference between those with a 'responsible' view and others. *Heavy* smokers in non-manual classes (and also own-account trades occupations) were, however, likely to reply yes to the 'own fault' question. The same was true of very *heavy* drinkers. Among women, smoking and drinking were consistently assoc-iated with 'internal' locus of control: it has, of course to be remembered that for women drinking is associated with higher occupational status or higher income within broad classes.

THE RELATIVE EFFECTS OF CIRCUMSTANCES AND ATTITUDES UPON BEHAVIOUR

It has been demonstrated that 'attitudes' – whether defined as a general positive orientation towards responsibility for health, or internal locus of control, or measured in terms of beliefs about the importance of specific behavioural factors for health – do appear to be associated with behaviour. In general, those who have positive attitudes or believe that behaviour is important are more likely to have 'healthy' lifestyles: this does depend on the behaviour being considered, however, and it has to be noted that there are many individuals for whom it is not true. As Chapter 6 demonstrated, personal characteristics and circumstances – income, education, family, region of residence – are also strongly associated with lifestyle habits. To what extent is the connection between attitudes and behaviour due to these intervening characteristics?

The method chosen here to illustrate these relative effects is that known as 'causal analysis', a simple method of using weighted marginal differences in cross-tabulations in order to construct partial correlations (Hellevik 1984). This involves setting up very general models, in which behaviour is, for instance, simply characterized as 'good' or 'bad', and requires assumptions to be made about the direction of causation. In the models which follow, it is assumed that, for instance, education 'causes' social class, or that attitudes to some degree 'cause' behaviour. Of course, it may be true that people's attitudes to smoking, say, are affected by their own smoking habits: some effects may run in the opposite directions to those being assumed. The models are simply 'what if' constructs. If it is presumed that things are, broadly, associated in this way, do the data support or refute this view?

The first examples are given in detail, in order to illustrate the method. Subsequently, the results of a large number of similar analyses are summarized. In each case, younger (18–39), mid-age (40–59) and older (60+) men and women were analysed separately, since the strength and sometimes even the direction of association may be different for each age-gender group.

Figure 7.3 illustrates the simplest model: higher social class 'affects' better diet, as do more positive attitudes. 'Attitudes' are defined here by high or low scores on the scale measuring the salience of diet as a health issue to the respondent. Social class and positive attitudes are, of course, associated.

Both the effects of class on attitude, and of attitude on diet, are shown to be positive and relatively strong in all age-gender

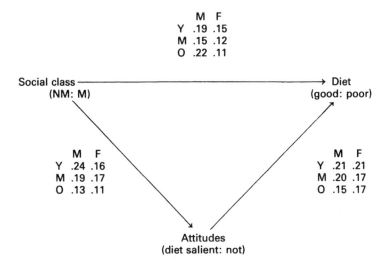

	Males Age			Females		
	18–39	40–59	60+	18–39	40–59	60+
(1) Bivariate 'effect' of class on diet, i.e. overall difference in proportions	.23	.19	.24	.18	.15	.12
(2) Effect of class through attitudes	.05	.04	.02	.03	.03	.02
(3) Direct effect of class controlling for attitudes	.19	.15	.22	.15	.12	.10
(4) Total causal effect	.24	.19	.24	.18	.15	.12
(5) Bivariate effect of attitudes on diet	.25	.24	.17	.21	.20	.19
(6) of which spurious association through prior variable class	.05	.04	.02	.03	.03	.02
	.20	.20	.15	.18	.17	.17

Figure 7.3 'Causal' analysis of the relationship between social class (non-manual: manual), attitudes to diet (diet a salient behaviour for health: not), and diet (good: poor)

groups, and strongest for the young. The effect of class on attitudes is rather weaker for young women than for men: this does not mean, of course, that women think diet less salient, but simply that the difference between non-manual and manual women is less. The effect of class is strengthened by an indirect effect through attitudes, but only to a small extent (in Figure 7.3 (2), .24 × .21, or .05 for the younger men), and least important for older people. About one fifth of the apparent class effect is due to attitudes for young men, but only one twelfth for older men. The effect of attitudes controlling for class (7) and of class controlling for attitudes (4) are about equal in weight, except for older men, among whom attitudes are less important.

Income is added to the model in Figure 7.4. Social class 'causes' high or low incomes, and it is hypothesized that a part of the non-attitude class effect in Figure 7.3 may be due to income: higher incomes have the effect of better diets. In the model postulated in Figure 7.4, high income does indeed 'cause' better diets, most strongly in middle age and with least effect in old age. Income also affects attitudes, within classes: a higher income leads to a greater awareness of the importance of diet, again most strongly in middle age. The effect of income, both directly and through attitudes, is in fact as great in the middle years as the total effect of class. For younger and older people, however, the class effect is accounted for more by attitudes.

Region is also held to be associated with diet, and it is true that in this survey those living above the conventional NW/SE divide were likely to have a poorer diet, with more fat, sugar and starch and less fruit, vegetables and brown bread. Class is, of course, associated with region, with a higher proportion of manual families in the North and West. In the model shown in Figure 7.5, the bivariate effect of attitudes on diet is still strong, and region is associated with attitude even within classes: diet is held to be of more importance in the South and East. Thus the regional effect on diet is reinforced to a small extent through regional and class-related attitudes. The total causal effect of region is of similar magnitude to the effect of income.

The ordering of the model has to change if education is used, since education (of the respondent) is obviously prior to the individual's social class. Figure 7.6 tests the hypothesis that education 'causes' social class (and the association is indeed

183

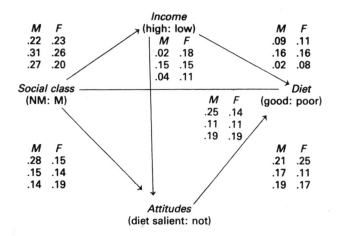

Figure 7.4 'Causal' analysis of the relationship between social class (non-manual: manual), household income (high:low), attitudes to diet (diet a salient behaviour for health:not), and diet (good:poor)

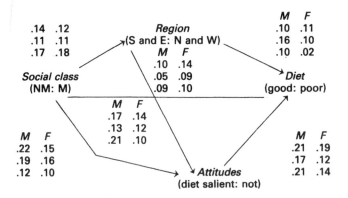

Figure 7.5 'Causal' analysis of the relationship between social class (non-manual:manual), region (S and E: N and W), attitudes to diet (diet a salient behaviour for health:not), and diet (good:poor)

shown to be very strong, though less for women than for men because of the method of categorizing married women), and, independently, affects attitudes. Here the total causal effect of education on dietary habits is shown to be strong, with the better educated having better diet. For men over 40 a large part

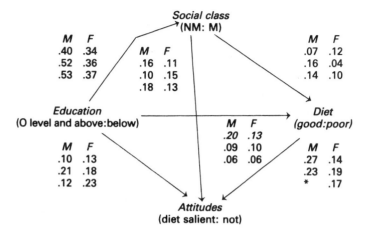

* low number

Figure 7.6 'Causal' analysis of the relationship between education (O level and above:below), social class (non-manual:manual), attitudes to diet (diet a salient behaviour for health:not), and diet (good:poor)

of this effect is through class and class-related attitudes, but for younger men and all women, education irrespective of class is more important.

Turning to exercise, non-manual class is still associated with more positive attitudes, though the difference between classes is less than that for diet, particularly for younger men and older women. For both men and women, attitudes are strongly related to exercise habits, viewed simply as a bivariate relationship. Analyses similar to those illustrated for diet demonstrate that a very large part of the apparent class-attitudes-behaviour link is in fact accounted for by income. For young men, class with income controlled has a negative effect: that is, those with high incomes in manual classes are more likely to have a high level of exercise than those with high incomes in non-manual classes.

Other, more general, variables can be substituted for the specific 'importance of diet/exercise' used above – internal/external locus of control, for instance, or 'degree of self-responsibility for health'. Since these correlate so closely with the measures of attitude to specific behaviours, the results are very similar: class differences in attitude 'affect' behaviour little;

education (particularly for diet) and income (particularly for exercise) are more important 'causes' of behaviour.

The other two health-related habits, smoking and alcohol consumption, are obviously likely to produce more confused results, since as shown in Table 7.8 positive attitudes to the importance of these behaviours for health tend to be associated with *unhealthy* behaviour. A causal model of the 'effect' of education shows that with the other variables controlled the effect of positive attitudes on smoking is negligible (or, for young men, negative). The salient effects are those of education, among young people, and of class within educational groups.

A model including income demonstrated that, within social classes and educational groups, higher income 'causes' more smoking among younger men. At the same time it 'causes' a greater likelihood of anti-smoking attitudes, thus reinforcing the negative association of attitudes and smoking. The effect of region – with smoking being more prevalent in the North and West – was shown to be almost entirely a class effect.

Modelling of the 'causes' of alcohol consumption produces a complex of relationships moving in different directions, and with very marked differences between age-gender groups. Attitudes are weakly or negatively associated with drinking, when class is controlled for. Within social classes, income 'causes' the greatest effect: those with higher incomes are more likely to be moderate or heavy drinkers.

Finally, a very general model is illustrated in Figure 7.7. In the class relationship with overall 'healthy' and 'unhealthy' behaviour (defined by selecting the 'best' and 'worst' categories of behaviour pattern, Figure 6.1), which is the more important: income, or attitudes defined as 'internal' or 'external' locus of control? At a bivariate level, internal locus of control is associated with 'healthy' behaviour, and non-manual class is associated with internal locus of control. The causal analysis shows, however, that within social classes and income groups, locus of control has a negligible effect on behaviour. The apparent effect of attitudes on behaviour is largely spurious, through the prior variables of social class and income. The total effect of social class is partly through income (one half or more for elderly men, and women in the middle years) and partly through other aspects of class such as education.

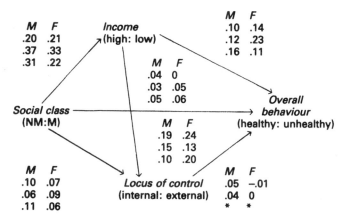

Figure 7.7 'Causal' analysis of the relationship between social class (non-manual: manual), household income (high: low), locus of control (internal: external) and overall behaviour (healthy: unhealthy)

Conclusion

To conclude that attitudes – however defined – have rather little effect upon behaviour if social circumstances are controlled for does not, of course, imply that the efforts of health educators to change beliefs or offer information are to be rejected as useless. Indeed, the importance of general education, as one of the components of social circumstance, is emphasized, and education must include health education – that is, receptivity to information and the opportunity to acquire accurate beliefs. *Within* social classes, education has been shown to have an independent effect upon 'healthy' behaviour. The fact that attitudes, controlling for education, have less of an effect must, however, suggest that it is not any attitudinal change which is important, but rather the complex of advantages which education provides.

Chapter Eight

BEHAVIOUR AND HEALTH

The analysis now returns to the patterns of behaviour illustrated in Figures 6.1–6.3. How are they related to health? The questions being asked here are not detailed epidemiological ones about, for instance, the disease associated with smoking or specific dietary habits. It is doubtful whether a survey such as this can add to this sort of knowledge. Rather evidence is being given about the association of 'healthy' and 'unhealthy' behaviour patterns, broadly defined, and health in general.

Here the problem of cause and effect emerges even more strongly than it did when the association of social circumstances and health was being examined. It may be hypothesized that voluntary lifestyles, as represented by exercise, diet, smoking and alcohol consumption, do affect health. Equally, however, health is likely to affect behaviour. Those with particular diseases may have been told to stop smoking or drinking alcohol, or to adopt a particular diet; those people who have conditions which limit mobility or energy are unlikely to take part in sporting activities.

Three broad groups may be considered: those people who said that they suffered from no chronic complaint or long-term physical impairment; those who did suffer from such a condition but said it had no effect whatsoever on their daily lives; and those with a chronic condition who said that it limited their activities in some way, even to a minor degree. The patterns of behaviour described in Chapter 6 (Figure 6.1) can then be examined to see if (controlling for age) they differ between the three groups. Whose behaviour appears to be a consequence of their health? It has already been noted that weight and sleep patterns are very different for those with, or without, a chronic disease, so that at this cross-sectional level of analysis neither can be regarded as always a cause, or always a consequence, of ill health.

In fact, proportions of people with the different behaviour patterns were almost identical for those with no disease, and those with 'non-limiting' disease. It does not seem – although of course there will be individual exceptions – that the conditions which people described as non-limiting had any effect upon the four behaviours. Those people with 'limiting' conditions were different, however. Notably, they took less exercise. To a lesser extent, they were more likely to be non-smokers. Thus, those with 'limiting' conditions were less likely than others to have behaviour profiles involving smoking, drinking, but high exercise.

Thus it appears that current behaviour is certainly to some extent dictated by the presence or absence of 'limiting' disease, but is not, on the whole, affected by conditions which were declared to be 'non-limiting'. For this reason, all the analyses which follow, relating behaviour to health (and, in Chapter 9, examining the interrelation of circumstances and behaviour as 'causes' of health status), are restricted to those people without limiting chronic disease. This device cannot altogether solve the problem of the direction of causation, but at least it makes more plausible the assumption that any excess ill health which is found may be causally associated with the behaviour concerned. What is being examined, then, is not smoking, or alcohol consumption, or diet, or exercise, as the cause of specific disease, but as factors which may be related to general ill health – which may of course be the symptom or the precursor of future disease, as yet unidentified.

Smoking and health

Of all four behavioural habits, smoking is the one which shows the clearest association with ill health of all kinds. Using the standardized health ratios of Chapter 4, the health profiles at various ages of non-smokers, occasional or very light smokers, and moderate or heavy smokers are shown in Figure 8.1. Since the effect of smoking upon measured lung function was very

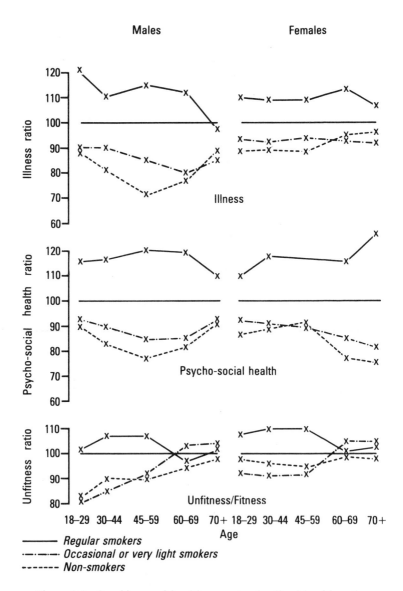

Figure 8.1 Smoking and health: age-standardized health ratios comparing regular smokers, occasional or very light smokers, and life-long non-(regular) smokers (note: ex-(regular) smokers are omitted) those without limiting disease only (all of a given age and gender = 100)

190

apparent (Table 8.1), and lung function is one of the elements of the fitness score, it is not surprising that *any* smoking appeared to depress fitness. (It is, perhaps, less expected that moderate/heavy smokers did not always have worse mean ratios than occasional smokers. For lung function alone, the difference, as shown in Table 8.1, was primarily a distinction between excellent respiratory health and that which was only good or average. For men over 60, smoking appeared to have little effect on health ratios. Remembering that only the non-diseased are being considered, with relatively low numbers in old age, it may be that a 'healthy survivor' effect is being demonstrated.)

Table 8.1 Smoking and respiratory function: per cent of smokers and non-smokers in different measured respiratory function categories*

Respiratory function	Males			Females		
	Age 18–39	40–59	60+	18–39	40–59	60+
Never-smokers						
Excellent	37	44	45	31	45	41
Good/acceptable	54	50	48	59	49	48
Fair/poor	9	7	6	10	5	6
(N=100%)	(440)	(143)	(62)	(683)	(422)	(323)
Ex-smokers						
Excellent	43	41	24	39	48	38
Good/acceptable	52	48	59	53	47	55
Fair/poor	5	11	17	8	6	6
(N=100%)	(168)	(232)	(235)	(256)	(200)	(148)
Pipe, cigar, and occasional or light cigarette smokers						
Excellent	40	32	24	22	39	31
Good/acceptable	51	56	54	62	52	62
Fair/poor	8	13	22	16	9	7
(N=100%)	(238)	(160)	(143)	(237)	(129)	(72)
Regular, moderate, or heavy cigarette smokers						
Excellent	25	19	17	21	20	18
Good/acceptable	65	67	59	68	68	64
Fair/poor	10	14	24	12	12	18
(N=100%)	(334)	(217)	(96)	(339)	(212)	(67)

* See Appendix B.

Smoking had, however, an even stronger and more regular association with the measure of illness. 'Cough' was one of the symptoms making up the illness score which smokers commonly declared. Of itself, however, this would not result in high illness scores: rather, smokers declared high rates of a wide variety of symptoms, especially among younger men and women. The association of smoking with psycho-social health is also notable. At every age, and among both men and women, those who smoked had higher rates of symptoms of malaise.

Ex-smokers and health

Ex-smokers – that is, those who used to be regular cigarette smokers who do not at present smoke at all – tended to be the unhealthiest of all. The fact that the health status of this group was worse than that of current smokers must obviously not be taken as suggesting that health deteriorates on giving up smoking: rather, those who give up smoking are likely to be in poor health. Almost 30 per cent of those people who had stopped smoking gave as their reason that they had been suffering ill health at the time of the decision. After the age of about 45, ex-smokers were more likely to have declared a chronic disease than either current smokers or those who had never smoked, and the more recent the decision to give up smoking, the greater the prevalence of chronic ill health. For instance, among men aged 45–59, 33 per cent of those who had given up smoking within the last 5 years said that they were suffering from a *limiting* chronic condition, compared with 16 per cent of those ex-smokers who gave up more than 5 years before.

It is therefore not surprising that the health ratios of ex-smokers are poorer, even when the analysis is confined to those who have no chronic disease. This is demonstrated for the dimension of fitness among men of two different age-groups in Figure 8.2. Those who have given up smoking within the last year are notably unfit. Those who gave up 1–5 years ago are less so. Those who stopped smoking 6 years ago or more are little different from non-smokers. This pattern applies also to the dimensions of illness and psycho-social ill health, though less clearly for older men and for women.

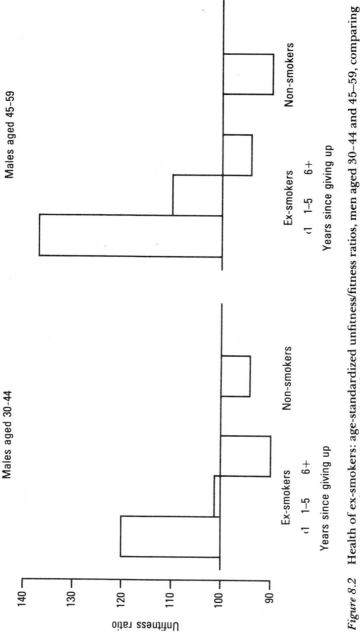

Figure 8.2 Health of ex-smokers: age-standardized unfitness/fitness ratios, men aged 30–44 and 45–59, comparing non-smokers and ex-smokers with different periods since giving up (all men of a given age = 100)

Alcohol consumption and health

The relationship of 'ordinary' rates of alcohol consumption to health was much less clear. As noted in Chapter 6, the number of respondents (especially women) who were ready to admit to addicted or problem drinking was relatively small, and many of these people are likely to be excluded from this analysis since they had a high probability of declaring chronic physical conditions also. (The health profiles of 'non-drinkers' are therefore unlikely to be distorted by the inclusion of 'abstinent alcoholics'.)

Very heavy drinkers, and also ex-drinkers, declared an excess of stomach trouble and indigestion (especially among the young) and liver trouble (especially among those in middle age). Male drinkers with an exceptionally heavy consumption also had high rates of hypertension. Among the 'non-diseased' population, however, how was alcohol consumption related to general levels of health?

For many age/sex groups, in specific dimensions of health, the most favourable health ratios were in fact associated with occasional or light drinking. For instance, age and sex standardized ratios for unfitness among middle-aged men may be compared: non-drinkers, 100; occasional or light drinkers, 89; moderate or heavy drinkers, 110. Among young men and women, drinkers were more fit than non-drinkers, though they did declare higher rates of illness. It seems likely that the personal characteristics associated with drinking (if the very heaviest, and already ill, drinkers are excluded) are more salient as predictors of health status than the drinking itself. Drinkers are, as noted in Chapter 6, more likely (especially among women and the elderly) to be of higher social class or to have higher incomes. Among younger men, they are more likely to have high levels of exercise. It would appear that these are the things which determine their health status, with the alcohol consumption itself having rather little effect.

Nevertheless, it may be that if very heavy drinkers are selected out – though this is a relatively small number of people – some effect upon health would be expected. Figure 8.3 shows health ratios for men whose alcohol consumption exceeded 50 units a week (there are insufficient women with a heavy level of admitted drinking for detailed analysis). These ratios are standardized not only for age within groups, but also for social class: that

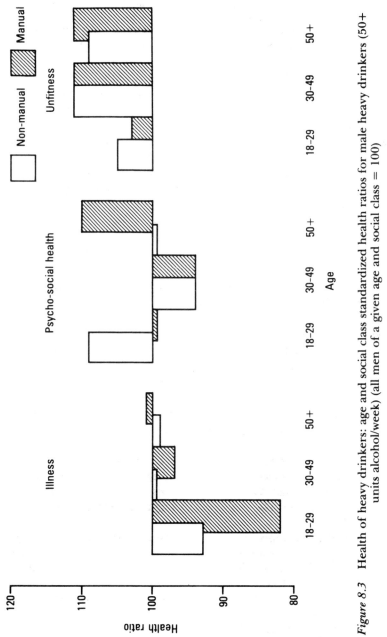

Figure 8.3   Health of heavy drinkers: age and social class standardized health ratios for male heavy drinkers (50+ units alcohol/week) (all men of a given age and social class = 100)

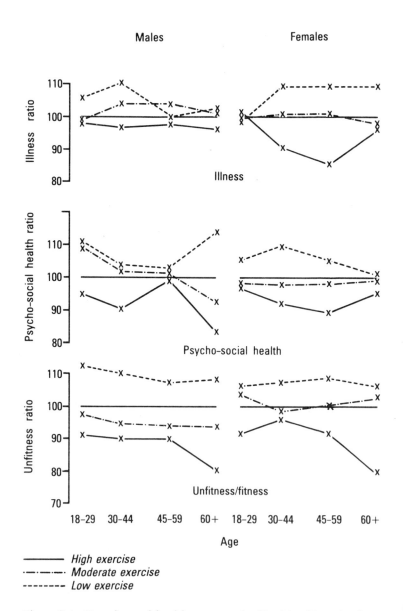

Figure 8.4 Exercise and health: age-standardized health ratios for those with 'high', 'moderate' and 'low' levels of exercise, those without limiting disease only (all of a given age and gender = 100)

is, the comparison is with peers in the same broad social class, so that the effect of drinking is isolated. These heavy drinkers still had ratios for illness that were favourable compared with the norm for their age/class, at all ages, or at worst only average. The youngest non-manual heavy drinkers had rather high rates of psycho-social ill health, as did heavy drinkers in manual classes over 50 years of age. Fitness ratios were rather poorer than the norm at all ages, however.

Exercise and health

For leisure exercise, the simple association with all aspects of health was very clear. Figure 8.4 demonstrates that, especially for men, the fitness ratios of those who engaged in a good or very good level of vigorous exercise were markedly better than those of the people who took little or no exercise. For most age/ sex groups even a moderate amount of exercise was associated with better than average fitness ratios.

The 'effect' of exercise upon psycho-social health was also marked, especially for older men. Associations with illness were rather less clear, though middle-aged women with high levels of exercise had particularly low illness ratios.

Diet and health

Again – and perhaps surprisingly – it was the dimension of psycho-social health which appeared to be most strongly associated with diet, measured crudely by the number of 'bad' dietary habits. As with the other aspects of lifestyle, it remains to be considered in Chapter 9 how much of this association is simply due to the social characteristics of those people whose diet is likely to be poor. Considering individual aspects of diet, it was shown (Cox et al. 1987) that greater fruit and salad consumption were clearly associated with less illness and psycho-social malaise, but social class and income are obviously likely to be intervening variables.

For the moment, it can be noted that the association of diet with illness and psycho-social health is strong at all ages, including the youngest; with fitness, less for the young (Figure 8.5).

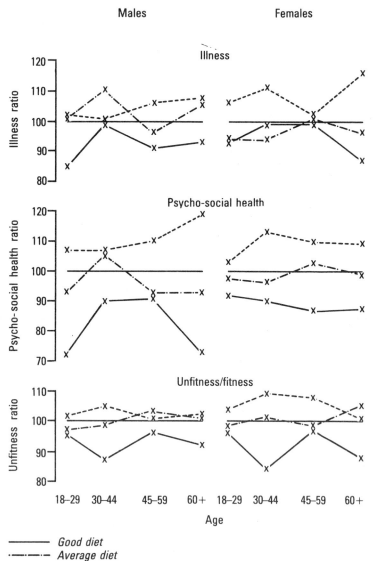

Figure 8.5 Diet and health: age-standardized health ratios for those with 'good', 'average' and 'poor' diets, those without limiting disease only (all of a given age and gender = 100)

BEHAVIOUR PATTERNS AND HEALTH

So far, aspects of lifestyle have been considered in isolation, and it has been established that – with the possible exception of alcohol consumption, below extremely heavy levels – each is clearly related to all aspects of health. The more interesting questions remain: what were the health profiles of those people with particular *patterns* of behaviour? Did it appear, for instance, that one 'healthy' behaviour could protect against the effects of otherwise 'unhealthy' lifestyles?

If those with all four 'good' habits are compared with those whose lifestyles were, in these respects, all 'bad' (Table 8.2) it is obvious that the health profiles of the two groups, completely standardized for age and gender, are very different. The lesser fitness of the 'bad' group, especially among young men, is notable. Even more notable, however, is the difference, at all ages, in psycho-social health: for both genders and at all ages those with unhealthy lifestyles scored very much more poorly. There is an anomaly, however, in the dimension of illness, especially among men. Men in the middle years showed the expected difference, but younger and older men with all four 'bad' behaviours did not declare high rates of illness.

Table 8.2 Standardized health ratios for those with all four 'good' behaviours and all four 'bad' (those without chronic disease only)

Health dimension	Males			Females		
	Age 18–39	40–59	60+	18–39	40–59	60+
All four health behaviours 'good': non-smoking, non-drinking, good diet, high exercise						
Illness	95	86	83	86	82	75
Psycho-social ill health	88	89	74	78	84	79
Unfitness	92	76	93	92	87	93
All four health behaviours 'bad': smoking, drinking, poor diet, low exercise						
Illness	91	124	93	108	99	*
Psycho-social ill health	127	120	130	116	136	*
Unfitness	131	114	109	112	116	*

* Small base number

To what extent might one 'unhealthy' behaviour depress health profiles? Comparing Table 8.3 with the profiles for those people whose four behaviours were all 'good', the ratios for those people with a poor diet, but who are non-smoking, non-drinking, with a high level of exercise, were very similar. A poor diet does appear, however, to be associated with greater illness with advancing age. Low exercise, even if the other aspects of lifestyle were healthy, meant poorer fitness at all ages, and generally poorer health in those over 60. For younger people, ratios for illness and psycho-social health were still favourable, however, especially among men. Alcohol consumption, even if diet and exercise were good, defined a group with poorer health among older women, more illness and malaise among younger women, and lower fitness among both men and women of middle age.

Table 8.3 Standardized ratios for groups with principally 'healthy' behaviour (those without chronic disease only)

	Males			Females		
Health dimension	Age 18–39	40–59	60+	18–39	40–59	60+
All healthy behaviours, except for poor diet						
Illness	73	89	109	76	87	98
Psycho-social ill health	87	79	76	95	82	72
Unfitness	86	92	94	77	92	92
All healthy behaviours, except for low exercise						
Illness	77	74	97	99	98	103
Psycho-social ill health	80	80	91	93	94	96
Unfitness	109	95	103	106	93	106
All healthy behaviours, except for moderate/heavy alcohol consumption						
Illness	93	92	96	100	81	114
Psycho-social ill health	91	88	81	105	81	90
Unfitness	83	101	91	82	107	100

To what extent might one 'good' behaviour protect? Among young men, those who were non-smokers had favourable health ratios – including fitness – even if they were heavy/moderate drinkers with a poor diet and low exercise. For the older groups of men, however, any favourable effect of non-smoking, in otherwise unhealthy lifestyles, was less clear (Table 8.4). It has to be remembered that, as noted in Chapter 6, this pattern of behaviour was more common among non-manual men than manual among the young, but showed no class bias among older men.

Table 8.4 Standardized ratios for groups with only one 'healthy' behaviour (those without chronic disease only)

Health dimension	Males		
	Age 18–39	40–59	60+
High exercise, but all other behaviours unhealthy			
Illness	106	107	*
Psycho-social ill health	120	118	*
Fitness	89	100	*
Non-smoking, but all other behaviours unhealthy			
Illness	81	96	122
Psycho-social ill health	86	129	157
Fitness	90	115	135

* Small base number

A quite common pattern among men under 60 (but not women or older men) included a high level of exercise, combined with smoking, drinking, and a poor diet. These men did have improved ratios for fitness, compared with those with low exercise. Their other health ratios were not improved, however: it is perhaps relevant here that this behaviour pattern was not differentiated by social class among younger men, and was most common at both extremes of the social class scale among men in the middle years.

Finally, the pattern of non-smoking and non-drinking among those with low exercise and a poor diet is examined, since it was (Figure 6.1) a common pattern in more elderly men and women. Young people in this group – rather few in number – had particularly poor ratios for fitness: as shown in Table 8.5, almost as poor as those for smokers *and* heavy drinkers with similar exercise and diet. Older men were also notably unfit. Mid-age and older women had relatively poor ratios for illness and psycho-social health, demonstrating again the strong relationship of diet and exercise for women with these more subjective aspects of health. The social characteristics of this group, described in Chapter 6, must be remembered, with their likelihood of lower incomes, lower education, and residence in industrial and rural areas.

Table 8.5   Standardized ratios for non-smokers and non-drinkers with poor diet and low exercise (those without chronic disease only)

Health dimension	Males Age 18–39	40–59	60+	Females 18–39	40–59	60+
Non-smokers, non-drinkers, with poor diet and low exercise						
Illness	105	95	96	86	121	120
Psycho-social ill health	102	87	102	99	111	112
Unfitness	123	101	140	115	100	89

Conclusion

Individual behaviours have certainly been shown to be associated with health. The association of smoking, or exercise, with fitness is not surprising. The strength of the relationship between behaviour and psycho-social health is less expected, though it must be remembered that one-way causation cannot be assumed: perhaps those who are depressed or anxious are likely to take little exercise, or to be careless about diet, or are likely to smoke and drink more.

Individual behaviours are also associated, however, with social circumstances (as shown in Chapter 6), and social circumstances are a strong predictor of health status (as shown in Chapter 5). It is therefore only to be expected that, when combinations of behaviour are considered, completely 'healthy' and completely 'unhealthy' lifestyles demonstrate very different associated health profiles.

Most people's behaviour is, however, mixed. Examination of different patterns shows that few generalizations can be made about the 'protective' effect of various combinations of behaviour. These effects often differ between the young and the old, or between men and women, and are commonly more clearly related to the social characteristics of the people who are most likely to display the particular behaviour pattern.

Thus a tentative conclusion can be reached: behavioural habits are certainly relevant to health, but perhaps less so than the social environment in which they are imbedded. This will be further examined in Chapter 9.

Chapter Nine

CIRCUMSTANCES, BEHAVIOUR, AND HEALTH

It has been demonstrated that economic and environmental circumstances, social well-being, and patterns of behaviour, are all associated with health. However, some of the important questions asked at the beginning of this volume remain – in particular, which of these things is the most important? The complexity of the relationships which have already been described must make it clear that an easy answer is unlikely.

Generalizations – that the health of those in non-manual classes is better than that of those in manual classes, that health is worse in the North than the South, that those who have a good diet are healthier than those who do not – can always be shown, at the population level, to be broadly true. But examined more closely, such generalizations must always be qualified. The young people in non-manual jobs in London who were shown to have such poor psycho-social health must be remembered, and the relatively prosperous men (and their wives) in the employers/managers class whose health was not as good as might, from their income level, be expected. The geographical question, in particular, is obviously complicated. In general (one exception being diet) there is more difference in typical lifestyles between types of 'small area' than there is between geographical regions. Patterns of behaviour by social class may be quite different in different types of area. Again, few generalizations are true throughout the life course. Different stages each show their own relationships. For the most part, both circumstances *and* behaviour have seemed to have greater impacts upon health in middle age, when compared to the young or to the old. People are less 'unequal' – though not completely equal – at the start of adult life, and there is convergence among those who survive to old age.

Thus the simple question – which is the more important, the environment or behaviour? – is probably impossible to answer, even when the possible dependence of behaviour on the social environment is left out of the equation. Some partial questions can, however, be asked. Health is clearly patterned by social class. Is it possible to estimate how much of this effect is due to economic circumstances, and how much to 'voluntary' lifestyles? How protective is 'healthy' behaviour, if circumstances are unfavourable? To what degree is 'unhealthy' behaviour damaging, in different circumstances? The social and economic environment, symbolized by the 'small area' analysis, has been shown to be associated both with health and with lifestyles – but are the combined effects invariate, no matter whether one lives in the North or the South, a city or a rural area? Individual situations of social support and integration, or troubled relationships and isolation, have been shown to be very strongly associated with the experience of physical ill health, as well as psychosocial malaise – but are these effects mitigated in any way by prosperity, or reinforced by poverty?

Circumstances or behaviour? Smoking, exercise and fitness

Among the four behaviours investigated, smoking and excessive drinking are obviously deleterious to health. The other two – diet and exercise – are rather different: they may be positive factors, promoting health, as well as behaviours which if neglected may do harm. This first example of possible relationships between circumstances and behaviour selects the effects of smoking for particular examination, since it is smoking which has been shown most clearly to be associated with poor health, especially in the dimension of fitness. Is exercise – also associated primarily with fitness – protective? Is it equally protective for all social classes?

Figure 9.1 compares, age-standardized in each broad social class, fitness/unfitness ratios for smokers aged 18–59 who took at least some vigorous exercise, and those who did not. In general, higher proportions of those in non-manual classes did take exercise, whether or not they were smokers, and smokers were

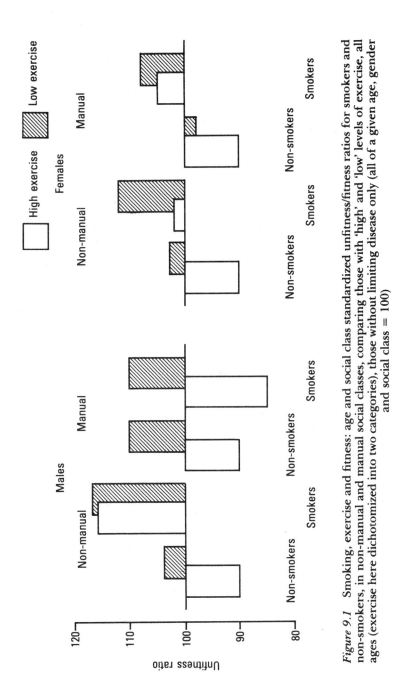

Figure 9.1 Smoking, exercise and fitness: age and social class standardized unfitness/fitness ratios for smokers and non-smokers, in non-manual and manual social classes, comparing those with 'high' and 'low' levels of exercise, all ages (exercise here dichotomized into two categories), those without limiting disease only (all of a given age, gender and social class = 100)

less likely to be in the high exercise group, whatever their class: this was shown in previous chapters. Manual men and women must be expected to have generally higher rates of unfitness, again as shown before. In Figure 9.1, however, the ratios are standardized within classes: that is, the norm to which the ratio refers is not only that for all men or women of a particular age, but also the norm for men and women of the respondent's class. Thus the 'effect' of the smoking/exercise combination is isolated, and easier to appreciate. The age group over 60 is omitted because at older ages there are too few smokers with a high level of exercise for the comparison to be made.

Of course smokers, in both social classes, had rather poorer fitness than non-smokers. Among non-manual men, however, the difference made by exercise was small. Among manual men, on the other hand, exercise made a considerable difference. Smokers with high levels of exercise had in fact particularly good fitness ratios, compared with all manual men, especially after the age of 40. Non-manual men who were smokers had poor ratios, compared with all non-manual men, even if their exercise was high.

Among women, class patterns were rather different. All smokers had poor ratios compared with non-smokers, and lack of exercise appeared to be associated with greater relative unfitness among non-manual than among manual women. Indeed, after the age of 40, manual women smokers who took exercise had fitness ratios little different from those who did not. Lack of exercise (and, probably, a poor diet, since these were shown in Chapter 6 to be strongly associated among women) combined with non-smoking (and, probably, non-drinking) was found to be a more characteristic behaviour pattern of semi-skilled and service workers, or housewives in poorer circumstances. It is thus possible that the effect of social circumstances, within classes, is modifying the effect of behaviour.

Nevertheless it appears, in this first example, that exercise *is* generally protective for the fitness of smokers. Smoking, of itself, makes rather more difference to the fitness of non-manual men and women than manual, but exercise is more protective, among men but not women, among the less socially advantaged.

Circumstances or behaviour? Exercise, work and fitness

Social class was used, in the preceding analysis, as a summary indicator of 'circumstances'. It is based, however, (for men) on occupation, and it may be profitable to look more closely at the nature of work. As Figure 9.2 shows (here considering only employed men, and using simple percentages of those who were of above or below an average range of fitness rather than ratios) the 'fit' were more likely to be sedentary workers than those whose work involved some manual effort, and those in heavy manual work were the least fit of all. (The categories are derived from self-reports of the physical effort involved in the respondent's own work, and may of course cross the boundaries of the conventional Registrar General 'non-manual/manual' distinction. Not all occupations classified as 'manual' in fact involve physical effort, and not all 'non-manual' jobs are entirely sedentary.) That 'heavy' workers should be more likely to be unfit seems counter to popular images of the benefits of muscular, perhaps outdoor, work, or the penalties of a sedentary life. It therefore seems of interest to consider whether behaviours – particularly smoking, heavy alcohol consumption, and leisure exercise – have any role.

Heavy workers were considerably more likely to be smokers, when compared with all other employed men (42 per cent regular smokers, compared with 29 per cent). They were only slightly more likely to be moderate or heavy drinkers, however (51 per cent compared with 48 per cent of all employed men). It therefore seems that smoking, though not drinking, may indeed be associated with their lower fitness. When smokers and non-smokers were compared, however, a similar finding emerged to that of the preceding section: smoking made a considerable difference to the fitness of those who were not heavy workers, but among heavy workers, non-smokers were little more likely than smokers to be fit.

What of exercise? It is usually suggested that it is leisure activity which is important for health, rather than activity at work. In Table 9.1 working men in the two age groups are divided into those who engaged in active sporting or other energetic leisure pursuits, those who took some exercise though not of a vigorous kind, and those who took little or no exercise at

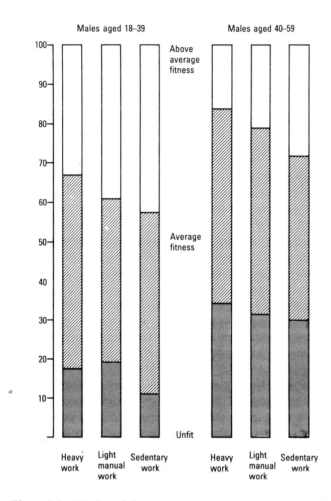

Figure 9.2 Work and fitness: percentage of males under 60 in sedentary, light manual, or heavy manual work who are of above average fitness, within an average range, or unfit

all. The fitness ratios of men who engaged in energetic sports were usually the best, whatever the nature of their work, but taking little or no leisure exercise made most difference for men in heavy manual work, rather than sedentary or light work, although the small group (only 39 individuals) of heavy manual workers of 40 and over who engaged in vigorous sports still had rather poor ratios. An unexplained anomaly is that sedentary workers who took no exercise were fitter, in both age groups, than those who took some – though always less fit than the sportsmen.

Table 9.1   Fitness ratios, standardized for age, of employed men by nature of work and level of leisure exercise

	Heavy manual work (N)		Some effort at work (N)		Sedentary work (N)	
Employed men age 18–39						
Engages in active sports	89	(108)	87	(161)	83	(87)
No sport, but a moderate level of leisure exercise	114	(91)	106	(99)	104	(65)
Little or no leisure exercise	118	(184)	106	(196)	98	(108)
Employed men age 40–59						
Engages in active sports	109	(39)	82	(56)	77	(45)
No sport, but a moderate level of leisure exercise	104	(105)	98	(132)	97	(71)
Little or no leisure exercise	107	(124)	102	(137)	88	(61)

(Standard: All men of a given age = 100. Note that employed men have slightly better than average fitness ratios, because of the poorer fitness of the unemployed and those outside the labour market.)

It seems, as far as fitness is concerned, that it is the occupations of heavy workers that are associated with unfitness. Obviously, it cannot be suggested, at the other extreme, that sedentary work promotes fitness: sedentary workers are more likely than the others to be of 'non-manual' social class, with the health advantage that this implies. But 'heavy' workers are not necessarily less skilled than other manual workers. The actual occupations of the men self-classified as heavy workers were examined: the most prominent occupation was that of construction worker, though many other jobs such as miners, agricultural workers, and transport workers, were also included. It must be assumed that a strongly adverse effect of the actual nature of these occupations is being shown.

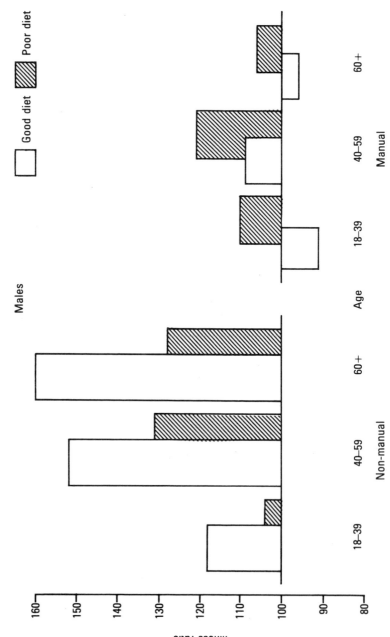

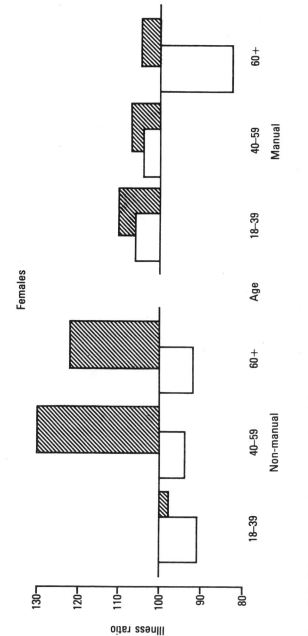

Figure 9.3 Diet as protective: age and social class standardized illness ratios for all those who are smokers and/or heavy drinkers, in non-manual and manual social classes, comparing those with good and with poor diets, those without limiting disease only (all of a given age, gender and social class = 100)

Circumstances or behaviour? Smoking, diet and illness

Smoking, and heavy drinking, were shown in Chapter 8 to be associated with high levels of illness symptoms, as with poorer fitness. Diet was an area of life also associated with illness. Smokers – though not necessarily drinkers – were also, of course, more likely to have poor diets. Not all smokers/drinkers have bad diets, however. If dietary practices are healthy, to what extent might this be protective? And is it equally so in all socio-economic circumstances?

Figure 9.3 selects all those who are smokers and/or heavy drinkers: the two habits frequently go together, of course, and there are rather few *heavy* drinkers who are not also smokers. In a similar way to Figure 9.1, illness ratios are shown for those who had good diets and those who had poor: older people are included here. Non-manual and manual men and women are compared, with the ratios standardized not only for age and sex but also for social class. The somewhat better ratios for manual men do not mean that manual men had less illness than non-manual, but that smokers were relatively less liable to high rates of illness in manual classes when compared with non-smokers: as shown in relation to fitness, smoking appeared to result in less depressed ratios for illness among manual men than among non-manual. Indeed, smokers with good diets among manual men – a rather small proportion of manual smokers – had lower than average illness ratios for the younger and older groups. *All* groups of non-manual smokers had relatively poor illness ratios, irrespective of diet, compared with the norm for non-manual men.

Moreover, in all age groups of non-manual men, the ratios for smokers/drinkers with a good diet were consistently poorer than for those with poor diets. Numbers are relatively small – 182 non-manual men with good diets, who are also smokers/drinkers – and explanations for the anomalous health of this group can only be speculative. The social characteristics of men, especially younger men, likely to show this behaviour pattern included high incomes and city or London areas of residence – groups among whom illness may be high irrespective of behaviour patterns.

Again, these relationships were different for women. Over 40, and particularly in the middle years, good or poor diet made more difference to illness experience of those in *non-manual* rather than manual families. As with exercise, a good diet did not appear to be protective for female smokers and/or heavy drinkers in manual social classes, except in the very small group of over 60s in this category. In contrast to men, non-manual smokers did not have an excess of illness, relative to all non-manual women, unless they combined this with a poor diet.

Circumstances or behaviour? Diet and exercise as protective

Finally, the analyses of Figures 9.1 and 9.3 are combined and summarized in Figure 9.4. Here, four groups of people are compared: smokers and/or heavy drinkers whose diet and exercise are poor, and smokers and/or drinkers whose good diet and exercise may be protective; those who neither smoke nor drink heavily whose diet and exercise are good, who may be expected to show the most favourable health ratios, and those who do not engage in the two 'bad' habits but otherwise, in the areas of diet and exercise, lead unhealthy lives. All ages under 60 are combined, and the health ratios completely standardized for age, since trends did not differ between the young and the middle-aged. Over 60, there were too few individuals in the group 'smokers and/or heavy drinkers with good diet and a high level of exercise' to enable a proper comparison to be made.

The combination of diet and exercise repeats, and indeed makes even clearer, the relationships already described. The obvious fact that those whose lifestyles are completely 'unhealthy' tend to experience more illness than those with no harmful areas of life has already been demonstrated (Table 8.5). Now, however, it is seen that if the social classes are distinguished – as a summary of socio-economic circumstances – there are notable differences. In the 'better' circumstances represented by non-manual class, poor diet plus low exercise had considerable effect, for both men and women, particularly among those with the 'bad' habits of smoking/drinking. Among manual respondents, however, diet and exercise were less 'protective' for smokers/drinkers, and indeed it was *non-smokers* with poor diet and low exercise who had the poorest illness ratios.

In Figure 9.5 this analysis is repeated for the dimension of

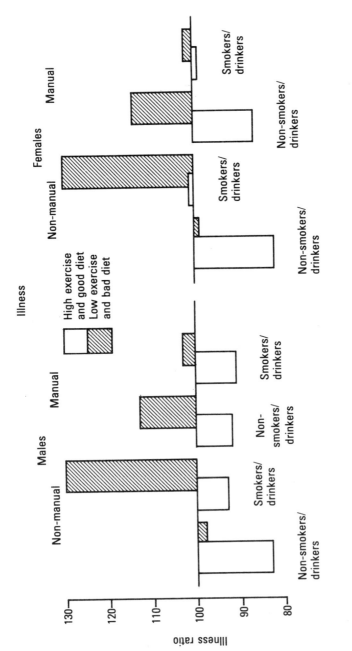

Figure 9.4 Exercise/diet as protective against illness for smokers and/or heavy drinkers: age-standardized illness ratios for those who are smokers/drinkers and those who are not, non-manual and manual social classes under age 60, showing the 'effect' of good diet and high exercise, those without limiting disease only (all of a given age and gender = 100)

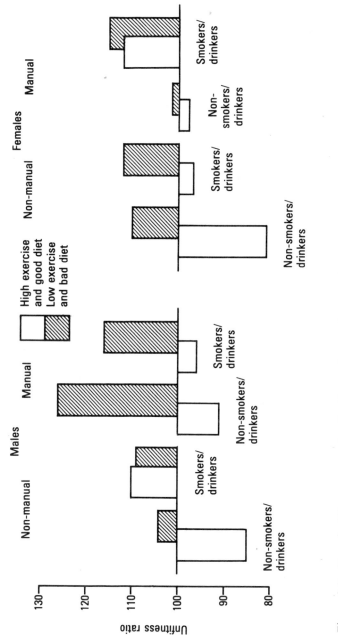

Figure 9.5 Exercise/diet as protective for fitness for smokers and/or heavy drinkers: age- and class-standardized ratios for those who are smokers/drinkers and those who are not, non-manual and manual social classes under age 60, showing the 'effect' of good diet and high exercise, those without limiting disease only (all of a given age, gender and social class = 100)

fitness/unfitness. Even for this more 'objective' measure of health, the same pattern appears, and, among manual men, *non-smokers* with otherwise 'unhealthy' lifestyles had the poorest fitness. Why should this be so? Each broad social class contains, of course, a wide range of social circumstances. It is in the manual classes, however, that the greater preponderance of severely disadvantaged circumstances is to be found – more of the unemployed, those with very low incomes. Smoking and heavy drinking are, other things being equal, associated with higher rather than lower incomes. It seems possible that the non-smoking, non-drinking, poor diet and exercise group in manual classes contains those in the worst socio-economic situations, whose abstention from the two 'bad' habits cannot compensate for the other unfavourable influences upon their health. If circumstances are good, 'healthy' behaviour appears to have a strong influence upon health. If they are bad, then behaviours make rather little difference.

Environment or behaviour? Regions and areas

Similar questions can be asked about the living environment, as summarized or symbolized by geographical areas and by the OPCS 'families'. What difference does a 'healthy' personal lifestyle make in a generally more healthy, or unhealthy, region of the country? Or in cities or industrial areas compared with rural areas, wherever geographically situated? And what difference does the individual's socio-economic position make in different types of area: does the above suggestion, that voluntary behaviours most affect health when personal socio-economic circumstances are favourable, remain true even when, for instance, the individual lives in an industrial area?

The aspect of lifestyle which was shown in Chapter 6 to be most strongly 'regional' is diet: it was noted there that although the educational aspect of social class had the strongest effect, and income, other things being equal, also had an effect, strong regional differences remained even if these were taken into account. Figure 9.6 therefore presents standardized illness ratios, in the two broad regions (North, and South and East) where differences are clearest, for those whose diet is good and those for whom it is poor. Women, rather than men, are used

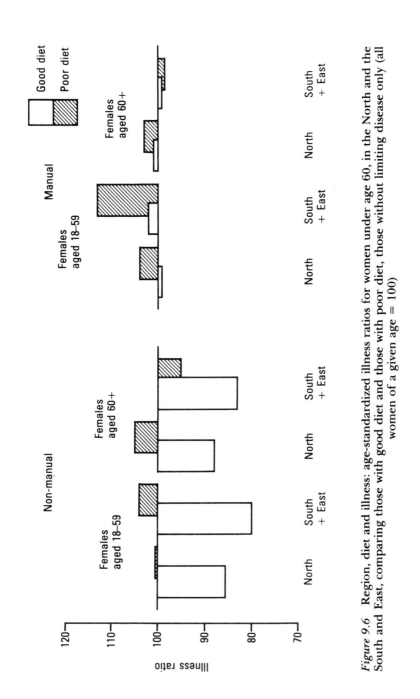

Figure 9.6 Region, diet and illness: age-standardized illness ratios for women under age 60, in the North and the South and East, comparing those with good diet and those with poor diet, those without limiting disease only (all women of a given age = 100)

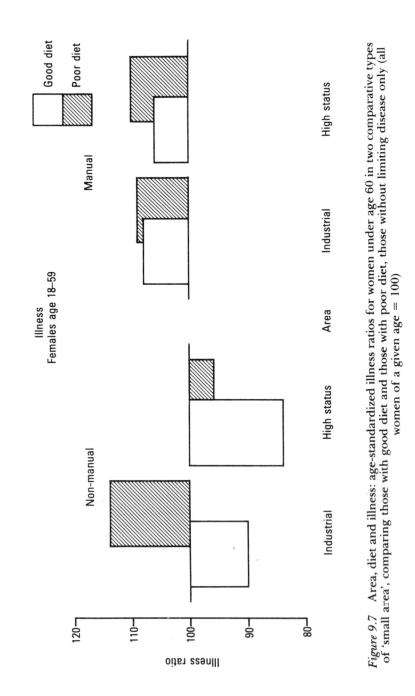

Figure 9.7 Area, diet and illness: age-standardized illness ratios for women under age 60 in two comparative types of 'small area', comparing those with good diet and those with poor diet, those without limiting disease only (all women of a given age = 100)

for the example since diet seems to be more important to women and more influential upon their health: because of the rather different patterns of association noted (p. 126) for those above, and below, the age of 60, these two age groups are separated.

The relationships shown are very similar to those of Figure 9.1 and 9.3. Whether in the North or the South, a good diet was associated with notably lower ratios for illness *only* among women in non-manual families. Diet made less difference to the illness ratios of women in manual families, and (below the age of 60) rather more for both broad social classes in the 'favourable' environment of the South than in the 'unfavourable' environment of the North.

Analysis by area families, rather than the 'North/South divide', produces comparable results (Figure 9.7). In industrial areas, wherever they are situated, illness tended to be high. A good diet was, however, protective for non-manual but not for manual women. Non-manual women with a poor diet had, in fact, higher illness ratios than manual. In high status areas – rather more likely, of course, to be found in the South – a good diet was associated with particularly low illness ratios among non-manual women. A poor diet increased illness, but it still remained at a better than average rate. Among manual women in high status areas, however, diet had little effect. Thus areas, and this aspect of lifestyle, were both important for the illness experience of non-manual women, but women in manual families were little affected by either.

Widening the analysis from only one aspect of lifestyle, diet, to generally 'healthy' or 'unhealthy' combinations of behaviour, a wider question can be asked: is behaviour equally protective against ill health in favourable living environments and in those areas where the poorest health is usually found? If one lives in a city or an industrial area, does individual behaviour matter more than if one lived in a healthier environment? And what difference do the individual's socio-economic circumstances make: is the vulnerability of the less prosperous reinforced in particular types of area?

An exploration of these questions was attempted by using broad social class as an indicator of socio-economic status, and selecting out those groups with 'entirely healthy' behaviour, or largely 'unhealthy' – i.e. those who smoke and/or drink heavily,

Table 9.2   Standardized health ratios for those in 'healthy' and 'unhealthy' behaviour categories in selected small areas, by social class (those without limiting chronic disease only)

Cities	Males		Females	
	Non-man.	*Man.*	*Non-man.*	*Man.*
Illness				
Healthy behaviour	100	82	96	71
Unhealthy behaviour	94	106	143	119
Psycho-social health				
Healthy behaviour	102	83	89	78
Unhealthy behaviour	108	127	114	137
Unfitness				
Healthy behaviour	54	98	78	89
Unhealthy behaviour	99	108	118	114
(N)	(29)	(27)	(58)	(39)
	(38)	(105)	(25)	(73)
Industrial				
Illness				
Healthy behaviour	102	83	89	78
Unhealthy behaviour	108	127	114	137
Psycho-social health				
Healthy behaviour	99	95	88	94
Unhealthy behaviour	120	130	128	126
Unfitness				
Healthy behaviour	105	86	87	110
Unhealthy behaviour	100	108	109	114
(N)	(46)	(34)	(72)	(71)
	(60)	(161)	(49)	(99)
High status				
Illness				
Healthy behaviour	80	102	73	106
Unhealthy behaviour	108	107	119	141
Psycho-social health				
Healthy behaviour	80	80	79	98
Unhealthy behaviour	123	115	111	148
Unfitness				
Healthy behaviour	87	106	86	103
Unhealthy behaviour	93	112	104	129
(N)	(55)	(34)	(111)	(64)
	(53)	(75)	(32)	(46)

and have poor diets, and take little exercise. Table 9.2 shows the health ratios for these groups in three types of 'small area' selected as examples – cities and service centres, manufacturing and industrial areas, and 'high status' areas. It must be noted that numbers, at this level, are sometimes small: there are, for instance, rather few men of either social class living in cities whose lifestyle is 'entirely healthy'.

However, there are some suggestive patterns. Wherever the respondent lived, it remained true for each dimension of health that non-manual men and women with 'unhealthy' behaviour had more ill health than manual men and women whose personal lifestyles were completely 'healthy'. This generalization apart, however, relationships are not the same in different types of area.

'High status' areas have been shown to be the living environments where the best health is most likely to be found: 'healthy' behaviour is also relatively more likely in these more favoured areas. Healthy behaviour, in a high status area, produced good ratios for all three dimensions of health for non-manual respondents. *Unhealthy* behaviour, in non-manual respondents, was associated, however, with considerably greater ill health, especially, among men, psycho-social malaise. (Fitness among nonmanual men was still better than average, however.) Among manual men and women, on the other hand, behaviour was not always so salient, and psycho-social health was the only dimension where healthy behaviour was associated with above-average health. Again, it seems that in high status areas individual behaviour is more important in non-manual classes among men but not so clearly among women.

Cities and service centres, and manufacturing and industrial areas, chosen as the areas where health is generally poorest, showed a different pattern. In these areas, 'healthy' or 'unhealthy' behaviour made little difference to the health ratios of non-manual men, who were shown in Chapter 6 to have rather poor health when compared with non-manual men in other areas. On the other hand, the relative health of manual men was particularly good if their behaviour was 'healthy' – indeed, their illness and psycho-social ill health were less than that of nonmanual men – but particularly poor if their behaviour was 'unhealthy'. These manual men with entirely healthy lifestyles were, of course, a minority in these unfavourable areas, where a pattern of smoking, drinking, and poor diet was more common. There seems to be some suggestion that they are a special and selected group.

Among women, the same group similarly tended to have particularly good health (except on the dimension of fitness in industrial areas). In contrast to men, however, behaviour tended to be salient among both broad social classes.

Socio-economic circumstances or social support?

The role of social support remains to be considered. It was suggested in Chapter 5 that psycho-social factors – stress, social activities, support, social integration – had to be seen as occupying an intermediate place between behavioural and socio-economic aspects of lifestyle. No matter how they are regarded, they were certainly shown to have a strong association with health. This was true not only of the psycho-social dimension of health – which would not be surprising – but also of physical health, especially the experience of illness.

Unfortunately for the individuals involved, stress, or lack of support, and other forms of social disadvantage frequently go together. People with very low incomes, the unemployed, single-handed parents, the divorced and separated, elderly widowed men living alone – all these fared badly on measures of stress and on measures of social isolation. Of course, at the individual level the association is not invariate: the wealthy may experience stress, and those in troubled social circumstances may still obtain support from their family, friends and community. Thus it is possible to ask: which is the more damaging, socio-economic disadvantage or deprivation in social relationships? Is the 'stress' described by those in advantageous economic circumstances as damaging as the stress described by the poor? In poor socio-economic circumstances, can a good level of social support be protective?

A simple representation of the associations between social support and illness and psycho-social health is shown in Figure 9.8. It has already been shown that social support is associated with these dimensions of health in both broad social classes (Figure 5.12). Here, household income, arbitrarily divided into 'low' and 'high' (with the division at £580/month), is used rather than social class. The measure of social support is the subjective scale described on p. 109. At all ages over 40, the relationships appeared to be patterned in a very similar way. For those under 40, however, they were rather different: two age-groups, 18–39 and 40 and over, are therefore distinguished.

For all age/gender groups except the young men, it is obvious that low income and lack of social support are each associated with high illness. Those who had low incomes had more illness, and these who lacked social support had more unfavourable ratios whether their incomes were high or low. For men and women over 40, support made more difference if income was low, and lack of support raised illness ratios only slightly if income was high. For these over-40s, income – or the occupational or social class variables associated with income – appeared to be more salient than social support: less illness was experienced by the high income, low support group than by those with high support but low income. Men under 40 were different, however: income made no difference as long as there was no lack of social support.

Very similar, though as would be expected more extreme, relationships were found with the dimension of psycho-social health. Social support showed a very strong effect, among men – but not women – more marked if income was low. For this aspect of health, high social support even with a low income was more favourable than a high income if support was felt to be lacking.

In order that some statistical estimate of the relative weights of social support and income could be made, with their interaction taken into account, the relationships described in Figure 9.8 were subjected to a series of loglinear analyses. Table 9.3 shows the resulting odds ratios. As Figure 9.8 suggested, for the dimension of illness, income had greater weight than social support for men and women over 40. Social support being equal, those with a low income had odds of nearly 1.5:1 of coming into the 'high illness' category. Social support also had an independent effect for men, however: income being equal, those men with a lack of social support had odds of 1.2:1 of having 'high' illness. Among young women, as Figure 9.8 suggested, social support had a greater effect than income.

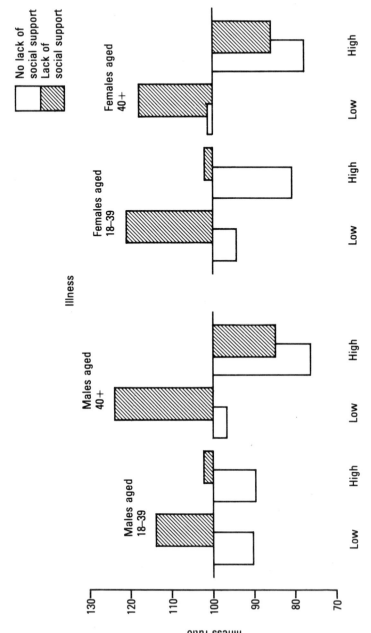

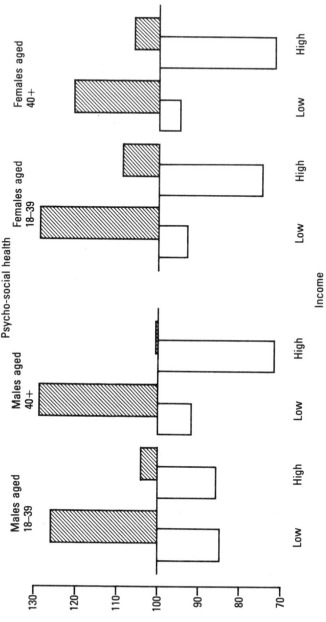

Figure 9.8 Social support, income and health: age-standardized ratios, illness and psycho-social health, for those with low and high household incomes (below and above £580/month), comparing those with no felt lack of social support and those with some lack, those without limiting disease only (all of a given age and gender = 100)

Table 9.3 Odds ratios (loglinear analysis): association of income and perceived social support with illness and psycho-social health

	Males		Females	
	Age 18–39	40+	18–39	40+
Odds of high level of illness				
Income – low: high	NS	1.45	1.20	1.42
Social support – no: yes	NS	1.21	1.45	NS
Interaction of income and social support	NS	NS	NS	NS
Odds of low level of psycho-social health				
Income – low: high	1.15	1.41	1.35	1.35
Social support – no: yes	1.48	1.26	1.52	1.52
Interaction of income and social support	NS	NS	NS	1.14

For psycho-social health, a low income increased the probability of high illness for both sexes and all ages, whatever the level of social support, though least for young men. For this dimension of health, however, social support had the greater effect, income being equal: young men had odds of nearly 1.5:1 of high illness if their social support was low, and women of all ages odds of over 1.5:1.

The interaction of social support and income was always positive for both illness and psycho-social health, though it reached significance only for malaise in the older women: that is, the effect of low income and lack of support combined was slightly greater than the effect of each alone.

The relative effects of income and the simple – and probably very inadequate – measure of 'stress' described on p. 104 were also examined. For the reasons given there, it is difficult to consider stress as a possible 'cause' of poor psycho-social health. The relationship of a self-defined perception of being under stress to the measure of illness is, however, of interest. This is illustrated in a similar way in Figure 9.9. Being 'under stress' was strongly associated with higher illness ratios, and more strongly (except perhaps among young women) for those with low incomes than those with high.

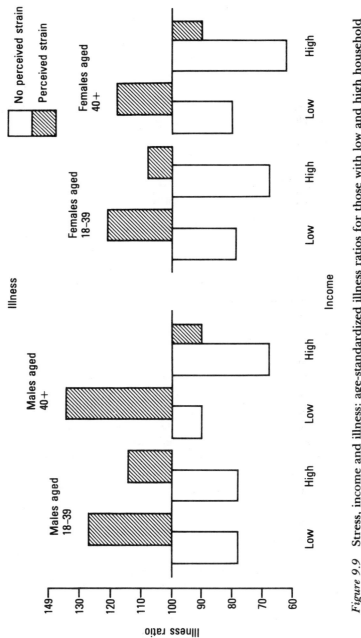

Figure 9.9 Stress, income and illness: age-standardized illness ratios for those with low and high household incomes, comparing those who do or do not feel 'under strain', those without limiting disease only (all of a given age and gender = 100)

Circumstances, social support or behaviour?

Social support, or a lack of perceived 'stress', are obviously protective against illness as well as against psycho-social malaise. It remains to be asked, however, whether these factors are more, or less, important than 'healthy' behaviour. Of course, behaviour may be associated with both stress and social support. Those who smoke or drink heavily may claim that this is because they are under stress, and social isolation may lead to unhealthy diets or lack of incentive or opportunity to enjoy leisure exercise. In fact, an examination of these relationships showed little overall association. Those who saw themselves as under stress, or felt a lack of social support, were a little more likely to engage in generally 'bad' rather than 'good' behaviour only among manual men between 40 and 59. For non-manual men, and all women, 'unhealthy' behaviour was not clearly associated with stress or social support, either positively or negatively. Some of those who were in stressed or troubled circumstances did lead unhealthy lives: equally however, some of those who led very integrated and socially active lives were smokers and drinkers with poor diets.

If social and economic circumstances are poor, however, how protective are social support on the one hand, or healthy behaviour on the other? Relevant socio-demographic groups will differ at various stages of life. For the young, 18–39, it was the unemployed, the divorced, separated and widowed, and single-handed parents of dependent children who were most likely to have high rates of illness and psycho-social malaise, and to feel that they lacked social support. Selecting the group with these personal situations, approximately 60 per cent of both men and women felt themselves to be lacking in social support. A majority of the young men fell into the 'bad' behaviour categories rather than the 'good', though the young women were more evenly divided. Thus numbers with *both* social support and 'healthy' behaviour were rather small. It appeared, however, that a combination of adequate social support and a lifestyle which included all four 'healthy' behaviours was indeed protective: this minority group had favourable ratios for both illness and psycho-social health. Either social support or 'healthy' behaviour appeared to have little protective effect on its own, however. Those who were disadvantaged on both counts had the poorest health record of all – for instance a mean illness ratio of 137 and a psycho-social malaise ratio of 144 for the 42 relevant young women – but the 35 young women with 'healthy' lifestyles but a lack of support fared little better with mean ratios of 123 and 140.

In the middle years of 40–59, the unemployed and all those not living with a spouse – whether divorced, widowed or remaining single – were selected as groups whose social situations had been shown in Chapter 5 to be associated with poor health. Numbers with 'entirely healthy' behaviour were again too small to examine any differential effect of social support in this group. Again, neither behaviour nor social support appeared to have much protective effect on its own, except for the dimension of fitness. Here, there was little difference between social support groups, but – confirming the usual greater association of behaviour and fitness in the middle years – those with 'good' behaviour were markedly more fit, even among these vulnerable groups. Their psycho-social malaise was no less, however, even if their behaviour was 'healthy'. As with the younger group, a *combination* of social support and healthy behaviour was, it appeared, protective – though less so for psycho-social health than for illness. Those who lacked social support and fell into the 'unhealthy' behaviour categories had particularly poor records of psycho-social health (e.g. a ratio of 159 for men).

To represent less favoured social circumstances over 60 years, those who were living alone were selected. Here, the associations were rather different. Social support or healthy behaviour, singly or in combination, had small protective effects, but the most notable association was the marked *adverse* effect of a combination of living alone, unhealthy lifestyle, and lack of social support. The small group of 40 men who came into this category had extremely poor ratios of 160 for illness and 237 for psycho-social malaise.

Thus, it seems that socio-economic circumstances, social support, and health-related behaviour all have independent effects upon the more subjective aspects of health, and all reinforce each other. If income and occupational status are high, behaviour is more likely to be healthy; if the confidence of social support, and the lack of a feeling of stress, are added, then chances of experiencing good health will be optimum. If disadvantaged circumstances, unhealthy behaviour and a lack of social support are combined, chances are at their worst. Even in poor circumstances, a combination of healthy behaviour and social support can be protective. In the absence of social support, however, little protective effect of behaviour could be discerned.

Conclusion

A broad conclusion must be, in this sample of the population and using these very simplified variables, that circumstances, including social support, have been shown to carry more weight for health outcomes than behaviour. It must be remembered that those who already have serious or 'limiting' disease are excluded: health is being defined simply in terms of 'everyday' health status, and nothing can be said about the development of future disease – which may well be related to particular behaviours – if it is not foreshadowed in the experience of poorer current health.

Although, as shown in Chapter 7, risk factors are certainly related to health, it does seem, however, that they are often more closely associated in good environments and social circumstances than in poor. Smoking made more difference to the fitness of men in non-manual social classes than in manual (Figure 9.1). Although this was not true of women, among whom smoking was associated with lower fitness equally in all social classes, there were other ways in which women's behaviour was more clearly related to their health in non-manual classes: for instance, exercise was more protective, and a poor diet made little difference to the fitness or illness of women in manual classes, whether or not they were smokers and/or drinkers (Figures 9.5, 9.6). A good diet made more difference for non-manual women in the favourable South than in the unfavourable North (Figure 9.6). For both genders, a good diet was most clearly associated with health in non-manual classes, and to exhibit all four 'unhealthy' behaviours meant notably poor health, relatively, for non-manual men and women (Figure 9.4).

On the other hand it must be noted that a good diet and high level of exercise were associated with lower illness and better fitness among manual men, especially if they were also non-smokers and non-drinkers (Figures 9.4, 9.5). Thus, while 'risk factors' certainly seemed to carry more weight in the more favourable circumstances, there was also some evidence of the 'protective' value of healthy behaviour, among men, in less favourable circumstances. It was among men also that lack of stress or an adequate level of social support were particularly protective for those with low incomes.

It might have been expected that this multiplicative effect – where lack of support and poverty reinforce each other to produce the worst effects on health – would be generally true of behaviour also. Are not those who are most vulnerable, because of their social, economic or geographical environment, likely to do most harm to their health if behavioural insults are added? At the extremes it is of course true that the worst health was found where poverty, an industrial or inner-city environment, disturbed social relationships, and a completely unhealthy pattern of behaviour, were all combined. For the majority of the population, however, circumstances are not extreme, and behaviour is rarely totally healthy or totally unhealthy. For this great majority, it seems that health is *primarily* affected by the environment, and by the characteristics – occupation, income, housing – subsumed under the broad description of 'social class'. It is among those who are not environmentally vulnerable that harmful behavioural habits such as smoking appear to produce a greater effect.

In some of the associations which have been shown, it is obvious that the relationship cannot be a causal one. For instance, a good diet cannot be thought to *cause* relatively more illness among non-manual men who are smokers and/or drinkers, nor are the particularly low illness ratios of manual women over 60 with a similar behaviour pattern likely to be a result of their smoking/drinking and dietary habits (Figure 9.3). This latter group of manual women are not typical of their age and class: they are likely to have higher incomes than other elderly manual women. The non-manual men who are smokers and/or heavy drinkers with a good diet are likely to be characterized by particular occupations (e.g. managerial rather than professional or clerical), areas of residence (including cities), and high incomes: their health has been shown before to be relatively poor, compared with other non-manual men. In other words, behavioural patterns distinguish groups which differ in many other ways. This is perhaps additional evidence that social circumstances, occupations, and 'lifestyles' defined in a broader sense than simply the measurement of smoking, alcohol consumption, diet and exercise have a greater weight than this restricted definition of healthy behaviour.

Chapter Ten

CONCLUSIONS AND POLICY IMPLICATIONS

A broad conclusion reached at the end of Chapter 9 was that 'circumstances' – not only socio-economic circumstances and the external environment, but also the individual's psycho-social environment – carry rather more weight, as determinants of health, than healthy or unhealthy behaviours. There is no doubt that the four behaviours examined, and in particular smoking, are relevant to health. They have most effect, however, when the social environment is good: rather less, if it is already unhealthy. Unhealthy behaviour does not reinforce disadvantage to the same extent as healthy behaviour increases advantage. This seems to suggest that the prior effect on health is the general lifestyle associated with economic or occupational position. Only in the more favourable circumstances is there 'room' for considerable damage or improvement by the adoption of voluntary health-related habits.

This may seem contrary to received wisdom. Because this, and some others of the findings of this analysis, are perhaps novel, care has been taken throughout to examine the evidence step by step, with the picture building up in each successive chapter. Chapter 5 showed that health – related to age and gender in the ways first demonstrated in Chapter 4 – is certainly associated with social and personal circumstances in ways which, because of the large sample of people available, can be shown to be very regular. Health, in all its dimensions, is associated with social class, with income, with personal living circumstances and with the wider environment. But perhaps this is only because those in particular social situations have typical patterns of health-related behaviour? To a somewhat lesser extent, it is true that those personal habits which are usually thought to have the most health-harming or health-promoting effect do mark out different groups of the population, as Chapter 6 demonstrated. Smoking, diet and exercise are certainly class-related. And patterns of behaviour are certainly, though not always straightforwardly, associated with health, as shown in Chapter 8. But perhaps – and here the argument becomes circular – this is only because these patterns are typical of the group whose circumstances have already singled them out as more, or less, likely to be healthy?

One important finding of this study has been that, in fact, few people's lifestyles are totally healthy or unhealthy: most are mixed. Only about 15 per cent of the sample were found to have 'healthy' habits in all the four areas of life examined, and only about 5 per cent had totally 'unhealthy' lives in these respects. Thus the effect of any one good or bad habit has to be considered in context, not in isolation. It is true that the minority whose lifestyles, judging from the limited criteria available here, are totally healthy, are likely to demonstrate health much better than the norm, and unhealthy habits will depress health markedly, even in favourable living circumstances. It is true that those who behave in totally unhealthy ways, and at the same time are subject to economic or social stress, were found to have the very worst health. The avoidance of behavioural risk factors was found, however, to be protective to only a small degree when involuntary lifestyles were unhealthy.

This is, of course, an over-simplified summary. The data which has been presented in this analysis is complex, and there has been no selection of that which might support a predetermined view, nor any exclusion of findings which are apparently contradictory. As a result, unexplained relationships abound: indeed, it may be that these offer the greatest contribution made by this data set, providing matters of detail for others to test, explore, and perhaps explain.

There are several firm conclusions, however: firstly, it has been shown that health is – as lay people clearly believe – multi-dimensional. Different groups or individuals can lay emphasis on different aspects or be unhealthy and healthy in different ways: circumstances and health-related habits can affect one dimension of health rather than another. In considering whether there are any practical or policy implications, therefore, this first point must be made: recipes for a healthier society must be clear about what they mean by 'health', and what aspect of health they are directed at.

A second conclusion is that there is clear evidence for social differentiation in everyday experience of health. It is not only in mortality rates, or in the distribution of specific disease conditions, that social classes differ. Indeed, variation in health more widely defined is probably greater. Differences in subjectively-experienced aspects of health – in the prevalence of common symptoms, in feelings of positive healthiness, in psycho-social well-being – are certainly greater than differences in objectively-measured physical fitness or the prevalence of diagnosed disease.

It has also been clearly shown that almost all the associations between social circumstances and health are strongest, especially for men, in the middle years of life. Some differences were apparent among even the youngest adults studied here, but commonly they were not great. Amongst older men and women, health became more 'equal' amongst those who survived to any given age. But in the 40s, 50s and 60s the accumulated effects of disadvantaged lives showed themselves most strongly.

Other important findings to which attention must be drawn relate to differences between men and women. Commonly, in health statistics women show less variation by social class than men (e.g. in mortality figures). It is possible that this is due to the use of 'husband's occupation' for the classification of married women, which – since their 'own' class may not be the same as their husbands's – may thus smooth out some of the variation between classes. For the most part, for the reasons outlined in Chapter 5, married women were similarly classified by their husband's occupation. For some attitudinal measures, there appeared to be less class variation among women than among men, and the use of education rather than social class to investigate these demonstrated that it was, indeed, probably an artefact of the classifying system. It must be noted, however, that even using the conventional husband's social class system, women's health did *not* appear to be less affected by social circumstances than men's. By 'own' occupation, the range of variation was very similar to that of men (Table 5.2). In many other instances women's health appeared to be *more* vulnerable to the social environment, especially in its more subjective dimensions: social class variation was greater in cities, or high status areas (Table 5.5), for instance, and young women were more affected than men by poor housing (Table 5.9). Women's diet was more affected by income (Table 6.10).

More interestingly, perhaps, it was certain relationships between social circumstances or behaviour and health which appeared to differ for women and men. Exercise appeared to be more protective for the fitness of male manual smokers than non-manual, and a good diet was not associated with less illness among non-manual men with otherwise unhealthy habits (Figures 9.1, 9.3). For women, these class relationships were reversed: exercise was not protective for manual smokers, and diet had more effect among non-manual than manual women. Area of residence impinged on health in different ways and behavioural patterns were not necessarily associated with area in the same manner (Tables 6.3, 5.7).

One of the more important conclusions of this analysis relates more generally to the effects of area of residence. In general, certain types of 'small area' (cities, industrial areas) were likely to demonstrate both worse health and less healthy behaviour than others (rural areas, high status areas): this is not surprising. Within small areas, however, class differences in health or in behaviour could be more or less marked: they were usually small in rural areas, for instance, and considerable in cities. They might even reverse: alcohol consumption was higher among non-manual than manual men in high status areas, but the reverse was true in industrial areas. The 'North/South divide' was shown to have limited significance of itself, and to be less important than type of area wherever geographically situated. This is the more notable, given the rather crude categories of area necessarily used here.

A conclusion must be that although broad statements about the effects of class or income or area of residence, or the relationship of behaviour to health, may seem to offer simple implications for policy, they can never be assumed to be universally applicable.

Social structure and inequality: causation or health selection

The evidence about social differentiation in health has been shown to be clear. The reasons why this systematic association between social position and health should exist are, however, as noted in Chapter 1, more problematic. It is from one point of view unfortunate that social class, as a composite indicator of advantage or disadvantage, has necessarily been used here as the principal summary measure of structural position. To say simply that classes differ does not readily suggest remedies for inequalities. The dilemma is that the objective of the study was to consider basic relationships within the population as a whole, not simply to identify especially vulnerable minorities: one result might be to conclude that the differences in health uncovered are the inevitable concommitant of societal structures, and thus not within the scope of practicable change.

Of course, *differences* in health are not the same as inequalities. Difference in health is not always related to class: there are healthy and unhealthy people in all classes and circumstances. The emphasis here on probabilities, on the likelihood of good or bad health, focuses attention on the way in which it is the expectation of good or poor health which is unequal – that is, on that part of differences which is related to social circumstances. It must be noted, however, that social factors will never 'explain' all of health.

The limited explanatory power of this study, as a snapshot of the population at one moment of time, must be acknowledged. There are, as noted in Chapter 1, two alternative hypotheses to explain class differences in health: one is that the environment has a direct effect upon health, and the other that the observed patterns are no more than a picture of the process of selection through social mobility: those who are healthy are more likely therefore to be prosperous, socially stable, occupationally successful, or geographically mobile to more favourable areas; those who are unhealthy are likely to fare badly. There is, of course, a great deal of evidence that much mobility – upwards and downwards – does take place in society, and the health of mobile people is usually found to be an intermediate compromise between that of their original class and the position which they achieve (Illsley 1986). Of itself, this might be compatible with either hypothesis. Only longitudinal studies, examining the whole life course, can properly examine these questions: certainly the Health and Lifestyle Survey is unable to do so.

It seems most likely that causal pathways lead in each direction. Throughout this study, care has been taken to note results which, in all probability, indicate that selective processes are in operation, at least in part – the higher likelihood of disease and disability among the non-married, for instance, or the poorer health of housewives when compared with women also working outside the home. Moreover, the sample was large enough to permit the device, used from Chapter 6 onwards, of excluding from the analysis all those with medical conditions which, they said, affected their lives in any way. The main purpose of this was to make it easier to examine the hypothesis that behaviour was a cause rather than a result of general health status, if consideration is confined to a population without serious disease. Also, however, it has the effect of excluding a high proportion of those who were downwardly mobile because of their health. Thus, although some of the associations of circumstances and health in Chapter 5 may be the result of selection, the conclusions about the relative effects of circumstances and voluntary lifestyles in the later chapters are less likely to be affected.

There is no evidence, however, about those who were *upwardly* mobile, who may have been selected by their good health to be, at the time of the survey, in favoured circumstances. One small test of this was made by selecting two groups by education and occupation. Those who left school at the minimum leaving age without qualifications but were nevertheless at the time of the survey in social classes I and II may be assumed to be the upwardly mobile, who have achieved more in occupational terms than might have been predicted from their start in life. Similarly, those who have A-levels or higher educational qualifications, but were employed in unskilled manual work, or were women married to unskilled workers, were assumed to be in an anomalous position and downwardly mobile in social class terms. The health ratios of each group were examined. Among the 385 individuals 'upwardly mobile' on these criteria, ratios standardized for age were little different from the norm, except that disease/disability was low. There were only 90 individuals defined as 'downwardly mobile', almost half of whom were women categorized by their husband's social class. Their fitness and disease ratios were average, but illness was high (a ratio of 114) for women but not men, and psycho-social health was particularly poor for both (ratios of 125 men and 135 women). This would seem to suggest that, using this very restricted definition of 'mobility', the absence of disease/disability may select for 'success', but lack of occupational success commensurate with educational status shows an effect upon the more subjective aspects of health.

If the evidence presented here can contribute only modestly to the debate about health selection, what does it offer which may help to explain – and so offer remedies for – direct social causation of ill health? There is some danger of seeming to suggest that if every individual were, firstly, wealthy, and secondly, happy (and the two are not of course by any means synonymous) all ill health would disappear: even to the extent that this is true, the policy implications are impractical.

However, attention has been drawn to particular groups, and particular forms of ill health, which may be more amenable to change. Some are already well known, and this study can do no more than emphasize their significance. Others are less obvious, and require further investigation: examples include the poor fitness of heavy manual workers, the poor health of younger non-manual workers in cities, the rather poor overall health of employers/managers in 'small' enterprises, the status as a risk group of elderly men living alone, the importance of social support in the middle years, the high illness rates of the young wives of unemployed men, and many other findings.

Perhaps more importantly, however, the wide view of 'health' which has been taken permits some consideration of *overall* susceptibility, rather than specific risk factors. The population studied here is (as in most industrialized societies) very sensitive to differences in socio-economic conditions. This sensitivity is general, and manifested in all dimensions of everyday health: it is not, as it once was, an overwhelming susceptibility to what used to be called the 'diseases of poverty'. Indeed, there are nowadays few diseases of poverty: the obvious candidates (infections, under-nutrition) have largely disappeared as causes of death, and the conditions which now account for most premature mortality (cancer, vascular disease, accidents, in the future perhaps AIDS) seem less obviously linked to extremely poor economic circumstances. It cannot be too strongly emphasized, however, that even for the conditions sometimes called diseases of affluence, because they have assumed particular importance in affluent societies, the disadvantage of the poor is greatest. For some of these diseases, there were once higher mortality rates in higher social classes. This is no longer true: there are now no major causes of mortality where death rates are not higher in lower social classes (Koskinen 1985, Blaxter 1986). A *general* susceptibility, clearly linked to socio-economic situation, is being demonstrated. As Marmot *et al.* have shown in the Whitehall Study of civil servants (Marmot *et al.* 1984, Marmot 1986) even for diseases with well-known specific risk factors (coronary heart disease and lung cancer) differential mortality rates between social groups cannot, largely, be explained by controlling for the risk factors involved. Increasingly it is being argued that differences in mortality are not due so much to differences in exposure to risk factors, as to differences in the resources available for coping with them (Antonovsky 1979). Psycho-social stress can be regarded as a general risk factor, and social support a coping resource. Low income is not necessarily associated with lack of social support, but it is the clearest 'marker' of exposure to other specific risk factors and lack of other resources.

Health behaviour and health education

What of more voluntary aspects of lifestyle? In the past, assumptions about cause and effect, and what is practical in terms of intervention, have been somewhat naïve. To identify behaviours – smoking, lack of exercise – as causes of ill health, and then to make sure that the public is aware of the facts, would – it is suggested – be enough to change behaviour. If those people with better education are more likely to follow this prescription, then this demonstrates only that the others are not behaving rationally, or do not have sufficient information: education is the answer.

The fallacies in this view have by now been well exposed. The Health and Lifestyle Survey adds to much existing evidence that beliefs are not very good predictors of behaviour. It seems from the interviews here that the public have, in general, learned very well the lessons of health education. They believe strongly that voluntary behaviours are the most important determinants of health. However, it is the better educated, and younger, who are more likely also to offer views about the importance of external, environmental and involuntary factors. Those who are most exposed to these adverse influences – those living in poverty, or with less 'healthy' work – are in fact *less* likely to attribute ill health to environmental factors, certainly in the context of their own lives. Moreover, it is those who indulge in unhealthy lifestyle habits who are *most* conscious of the links between behaviour and disease.

The questions of the valuation placed on health, and 'passive/active', 'negative/positive', or 'external/internal' attitudes to health, are obviously complex. Substantial proportions of the population did not see health as the most important thing in life – and these were more likely to be people with more, rather than less, education. Also, one *dimension* of this complex thing called health may well be valued over another. The notion of 'health as a value' obscures its multi-dimensional nature. It was clear from their descriptions that many people were aware that trade-offs between different aspects might have to be made.

It is also clear that many people do lead healthy lives without necessarily having health promotion as their motivation. Equally, 'unhealthy' habits may be seen as determined by other considerations besides health. The apparent contradiction between beliefs which are expressed when the individual is forced by an interviewer's questioning to consider what he or she thinks, and the details of what he or she does in terms of actual everyday behaviour, is thus easy to understand.

Also, different aspects of behaviour must be considered separately. It has commonly been shown that there are only modest associations between one type of health-related behaviour and another: the avoidance of health-damaging behaviours, and the practice of health-promoting behaviours, may be differently related to other aspects of lifestyle. As Chapter 6 indicated, the entirely heedless or the entirely health-oriented are only small minorities among the population. An issue which

241

this survey cannot address, but which is also relevant, is the stability of behaviour patterns over time: others have produced some evidence that it is not in fact very high.

It can be suggested that there were two groups in this survey among whom a lack of positive attitudes and unhealthy behaviour could be associated. One contained men and women – more men, and likely to be young – who did not appear to think about health at all. They might be well aware of public health issues, but did not see any relevance to their own lives. There was a strong probability that they would call their own health 'good', even if other evidence suggested it was less than perfect. Some of this group were wealthy, but more were in lower-income groups. These people were likely to combine smoking, drinking and a poor diet, though they might – for reasons of pleasure or achievement, not health – take an adequate amount of exercise.

The second group was entirely different. These were much concerned about health, and had many ideas about it. They were more likely to be women, and older, and in poor health. They were also likely to be in troubled social circumstances and to have low incomes. Their attitudes were fatalistic: health was, as a general principle, the consequence of behaviour, but this did not apply to them; health was extremely important, but they themselves had no control over it. These people were also likely to have very unhealthy habits, with the possible exception of heavy drinking.

Obviously, the relationships between values, attitudes and behaviour are very different for these two groups. Both might be said to 'need' health education, but not of the same kind: the first might be 'taught' to value health, and the second helped to see that they could be more demanding consumers of both illness-managing and health-promoting services.

For the majority, however, the potential benefits of health education are not altogether straightforward. Not all heavy-drinking, smoking, totally health-careless individuals are in disadvantaged circumstances, of course, but those who are prosperous and well-educated who behave in this way are minorities. They certainly harm their health, but there can be no assumption that changing their behaviour, if it were possible, would improve their health to the majority level: they are by definition different. (There has been some suggestion that such anomalous groups are characterized by, for instance, combinations of occupation and area of residence.) Similarly, those who are in health-damaging circumstances – whether economic or in their personal social situations – who behave in very health-conscious ways are rather special minorities, and it cannot be assumed either that it is practicable to expect the majority of people in these circumstances to follow their example, or that the health effects would be similar. Obviously, it is not being suggested that the fitness of a low-income unskilled worker or his wife living in an inner city would not be improved if he or she did not smoke. But the improvement would be modest: their health would still be poorer than the average.

In any case, the scope for personal change in behaviour depends on the availability of resources for change. 'Education' aimed at the personal modification of lifestyles may be resisted if the power to change is, or is felt to be, unavailable. The ability to choose is inevitably restricted by living and working conditions. The ideology which places the responsibility for health squarely upon the individual him- or herself may, indeed, be counter-productive. That health has a moral connotation is not of course new: the equation of health with virtue was not invented by contemporary health education, which only reinforces a very deep-seated concept. Nevertheless disdain for the weak or unfortunate as morally reprehensible is not an attractive attitude to promulgate. The apologetic air with which those who were not healthy spoke about their health was a pervasive impression, even in this largely structured survey.

The evidence here, as elsewhere, suggests that education is certainly relevant, but more because better education is associated with general differences in patterns of life than because discrete parts of a lifestyle can be changed. Health-change policies which focus entirely on the individual may be ineffective not only because exposure to health risks is largely involuntary, but also, as this study has shown, because of unwarranted assumptions about the extent to which behaviour can, in these circumstances, be effective in improving health.

APPENDICES

(Note: only a selection of the questions in the Health and Lifestyle Survey are listed, i.e. those which were used for the formation of the indices used in this analysis.)

A. Health: questions, measurements, and the formation of indices

Disease/disability

Q.21 a Do you have any longstanding illness, disability or infirmity?

b (if yes) What is the matter with you? (open-ended)

c Does it limit your activities in any way compared with people of your own age? (yes/no)

d (if yes) How does it affect you? Do you have to take special care some of the time? (yes/no)

e Are you limited in the amount of work or the kind of work you can do, or in your social life? (yes/no)

f Are you able to work (or do housework)? (yes/no)

g Can you climb stairs? (yes/no)

h Can you walk outside without help or aids? (yes/no)

i (if no) Can you walk around the house (flat) without help or aids? (yes/no)

j Do you have to have help with things like dressing or feeding? (yes/no)

Comments and notes of medication taken, made by the nurse conducting the physiological measurements, also taken into account in the identification of disease and disability.

Q.22 a Have you ever had (18 conditions named individually: asthma, chronic bronchitis, other chest trouble, diabetes, stomach or digestive disorders, piles or haemorrhoids, liver trouble, rheumatic trouble or arthritis, heart trouble, lung cancer, other cancer, severe depression or other nervous illness, varicose veins, high blood pressure, stroke, migraine, back trouble, epilepsy or fits)? (yes/no)

b (if yes) has it ever been treated by a doctor or hospital? (yes/no)

244

Illness and psycho-social health

Q.23 Within the last month have you suffered from any problems with (21 physical or psycho-social conditions named individually: headache, hay fever, difficulty sleeping, constipation, trouble with eyes, a bad back, nerves, colds and flu, trouble with feet, always feeling tired, kidney or bladder trouble, painful joints, difficulty concentrating, palpitations or breathlessness, trouble with ears, worrying over every little thing, indigestion or other stomach trouble, sinus trouble or catarrh, persistent cough, faints or dizziness, (F < 60 years) trouble with periods or the menopause)? (yes/no)

Q.24 How often do you feel under so much strain that your health is likely to suffer? (always/often/sometimes/never)

Fitness

Measured body mass index:
Height measured without shoes using a stadiometer, weight measured using portable electronic scales with an estimate of the weight of clothing, used to calculate body mass index: weight (kg) divided by height (m) squared. Using this index, four categories derived:

	males	females
Underweight	<20.0	<18.6
Acceptable/normal	20.1–25.0	18.7–23.8
Mildly overweight	25.1–29.9	23.9–28.5
Obese	>30.0	>28.6

Measured blood pressure:
An automated device used to measure blood pressure (4 readings) from which categories were derived:

Normotensive	<140/90 mmHg
Borderline	141/91–159/94 mmHg
Hypertensive	>160/95 mmHg

(Those under active treatment for hypertension included as hypertensive.)

Respiratory function:
FEV_1, PEF and FVC measured by an electronic spirometer. Categories derived using simple regression equations which give predicted values of FEV_1 and FVC, taking into account sex, age and height (see Cox *et al.* 1987). Those with transitory respiratory problems (colds, etc.) excluded.

Excellent	Equal to or in excess of predicted value
Acceptable	< 2 S.D. below predicted value
Fair/Poor	2 < 4 S.D. below predicted value
Very Poor	4 + S.D. below predicted value, or unable to perform tests because of chronic respiratory problem.

Formation and interpretation of health indices

Using the questions and measurements listed above, each individual was allocated a position on a scale 1–6 for each dimension of health:

Disease (1) no disease, (2) non-limiting disease, (3) 'has to take care', (4) limited in activity or mobility, (5) unable to work or unable to walk outdoors, (6) unable to walk indoors or requiring help with activities of daily living.

Illness 16 symptoms each scored 0 or 1. (1) score 0, (2) score 1, (3) score 2, (4) score 3–4, (5) score 5–8, (6) score 9+

Psycho-social health 5 symptoms each scored 0 or 1, Q.24 scored 0–3. (1) score 0, (2) score 1, (3) score 2, (4) score 3, (5) score 4–5, (6) score 6+

Unfitness/fitness Mildly overweight scored 1, underweight scored 2, obese scored 4; borderline hypertension scored 1, hypertensive scored 6; acceptable lung function scored 1, fair to poor scored 3, very poor scored 6.

(1) Score 0, (2) score 1, (3) score 2, (4) score 3, (5) score 4–5, (6) score 6+ (note that the scoring ensures that those who are obese, hypertensive, or with poor lung function, are placed in an 'unfit' category.)

In their 'raw' state the scores (e.g. 0–16 symptoms of illness) had, of course, very differently shaped distributions for the four dimensions. The conversion of each into a scale of 1–6 enabled approximately normal distributions to be obtained so that the scales could be more easily compared. It should be noted, however, that one of the scales, that applying to disease, is inevitably still highly skewed (with over 50 per cent scoring 1): this should be borne in mind when positions on the different dimensions are compared.

In forming the overall health categories (p. 54) and sometimes in discussions of simple classifications (e.g. the distinction between the 'fit' and 'unfit', p. 208) the scales are used to distinguish three levels of health: 'good' (1,2); 'within an average range' (3,4); and 'poor' (5,6).

To form the health indices (p. 49), more usually employed throughout for the comparison of groups of the population, each score was converted to an index by dividing by the mean value of the score for the population or for an age/gender group. When subgroups of the population were considered, mean indices were corrected by direct proportion to control for attributes (usually age and sex composition) of the group when compared with the population.

Errors have not been ascribed to the mean indices. They are obviously complex due to the limited number of classes in the original scaling and the proportional adjustments made to the means. The coefficients of variation of the unadjusted scaled values within subclasses usually varied around 30 per cent. These are obviously unaffected by the primary indexation but they could be reduced or augmented when corrections were applied to control for the age and sex composition of groups. Errors attached to means in subgroups are inversely proportional to the square root of the number in the subgroup, which suggests that where numbers are greater than 100 the standard errors of mean indices are likely to be less than 3 percentage units.

B. Social integration and support: questions and measures

Social integration

Score based on marital status, household (i.e. whether living alone), employment status, existence of children, existence of surviving parents, and answers to questions:

Q.9 a How long have you lived in this area? (Replies categorized into < 5 years, 5+ years)
   b Were you born in this area? (yes/no)

Q.10 Do you feel part of the community (yes/no)

Q.11a–f In the past two weeks how many times have you gone out to visit family, had family to visit you, had contact with family by phone or letter; gone out to visit friends, had friends to visit you, had contact with friends by phone or letter? (Replies categorized into low, medium and high contact for family and for friends)

Q.75 Have you done this activity in the past fortnight?
(Selected from a range of activities):
Community, social or voluntary work (yes/no)
Been to a church or other place of worship (yes/no)

Each positive item was scored as 1, with the exception of marital status, household, and contact with family and friends, which were weighted (married, not living alone, scored as 2, and Q.11 scored 0–2 for low, medium or high contact with friends). The resultant score of 0–16 was divided into arbitrary categories: very low 0–3, low 4–7, medium 8–10, high 11–12, very high 13–16.

Perceived social support

Score based on series of seven questions:

Q.12a–g Here are some comments people have made about their family. I'd like you to say how far each statement is true for you:
   There are members of my family (if no family, friends) who – make me feel loved, do things to make me happy, can be relied on no matter what happens, would see I am taken care of if I needed to be, accept me just as I am, make me feel an important part of their lives, give me support and encouragement (not true/partly true/certainly true)

Each 'certainly true' answer was scored 2 and each 'partly true' answer 1. The resultant scores were heavily skewed, with approximately 60 per cent of the sample gaining the maximum ('no lack of support'). A further 25 per cent scored 18–20 ('some lack of support') and 15 per cent 0–17 ('considerable lack of support').

C. Behaviour: questions and the formation of indices

Smoking

Q.55 Do you regularly smoke cigarettes, that is do you regularly smoke at least one cigarette a day (yes/no)

   b (if no) Do you smoke cigarettes, but fewer than one a day? (yes/no)

   c (and) Have you ever smoked at least one cigarette a day for as long as six months? (yes/no)

Q.56 a (if yes) How many cigarettes do you generally smoke in a day? (number)

(Also questions on cigar and pipe smoking, and a wide range of questions on past smoking, starting smoking, giving up smoking and reasons for it, etc.).

The smoking categories used (e.g. Table 6.1) are:

1. Non (current) smoker
2. Pipe or cigar smoker
3. Occasional cigarette smoker – < 1/day
4. Light regular cigarette smoker – 1–5/day
5. Moderate regular cigarette smoker – 6–19/day
6. Heavy regular cigarette smoker – 20+/day

Alcohol consumption

Q.47 a Would you say that you are a non-drinker/very special occasions drinker/occasional drinker/regular drinker?

Q.48 a (if occasional or regular) Would you say you are a light/moderate/heavy drinker?

Q.49 d Have you had any alcoholic drinks during the past week?

   c (if yes) (Respondent taken through 'last week's' drinking diary, noting amount of alcohol, type of drinks, time of day of consumption).

Q.50 Was this last week's drinking reasonably typical of your usual pattern/rather less than usual/rather more than usual?

(Also questions on past drinking, cutting down, reason for giving up or cutting down, and a range of questions designed to identify 'problem' drinkers).

The drinking categories used (e.g. Table 6.4) are:

1. Non (current) drinker
2. Very occasional drinker
3. Says regular drinker, but none 'last week'
4. Light drinker – says regular drinker, consumption 'last week' males 1–10 units alcohol, females 1–5 units
5. Moderate drinker – says regular drinker, consumption 'last week' males 11–50 units, females 6–35 units
6. Heavy drinker – says regular drinker, consumption 'last week' males >50 units, females >35 units

Exercise

Q.69 a On weekdays (working days) when not at work, how much time on average per day do you spend walking: to work, shopping, walking the dog, for pleasure and so on?

b (repeated for weekends or rest days)

Q.71 a In the last 7 days, have you done any gardening?

b (if yes) How much time overall did you spend gardening?

c Did any of this gardening make you out of breath?

Q.72 a In the last 7 days, have you done any DIY (explanatory elaboration)?

b (if yes) How much time overall did you spend on DIY?

c Did any of this DIY make you out of breath?

Q.73 In the last fortnight have you done any of (list of 17 sports, keep-fit and other vigorous activities, followed by 'any other physical activities')? How many times; average length of time each done; did activity make you out of breath?
(Also questions about physical activity at work, housework, general social activities, etc.)

Two categories of walking/gardening/DIY (combined) exercise were derived, based on reported duration, and 3 categories of sports/keep-fit/other vigorous activities ('vigorous exercise'), based on a typical energy expenditure of the activity and its duration.

The exercise categories used (e.g. Table 6.6) are:

1. High level of vigorous exercise (estimated energy output >2500 kcal/fortnight)

2. Moderate level of vigorous exercise (estimated energy output 1000<2500 kcal/fortnight)

3. Low level, but some, vigorous exercise (All the above might also include walking/gardening/DIY)

4. High level of walking/gardening/DIY (>7 hours/week) but no vigorous exercise

5. Some walking/gardening/DIY (2<7 hours/week) but no vigorous exercise

6. Little or no leisure activity of any kind

In analyses where 'high' and 'low' exercise are distinguished, the division is between categories (1, 2, 3, 4) and (5, 6). In analyses where 'vigorous' exercise is distinguished, the division is between categories (1, 2, 3) and (4, 5, 6).

Diet

From a wide variety of questions about specific foods and eating habits, including a list of 30 foods with the request to say how often each was eaten, seven items were selected (see Chapter 6) which clustered as the best markers of a nutritionally approved diet:

Q.37 How often do you eat fried food (not counting chips)? (answers dichotomized for the present purpose, less than twice a week/twice a week or more often)

Q.38 What sort(s) of bread do you eat? (answers dichotomized, granary, wheatmeal, wholemeal, brown/white and other)

Q.40 Do you usually spread soft margarine, hard margarine or butter on bread? (answers dichotomized, soft margarine/other)

Q.46 (part) How often do you eat:
Fresh fruit in summer? (answers dichotomized, once a day/less)
Salads or raw vegetables in winter? (answers dichotomized, once a week/less)
Chips? (Answers dichotomized, not more than twice a week/more than twice a week)
Sweets/chocolates/biscuits? (answers dichotomized, less than once a day/once a day or more)

In analyses where 'good', 'average' and 'poor' diets are distinguished:

good   5 + good food habits
average   3 or 4 good food habits
poor   0, 1 or 2 good food habits

In analyses where 'good' and 'poor' diets are distinguished, the division is made at 4 good habits.

D. Attitudes: questions and measures

Concept of health for another

Q.4 a Think of someone you know who is very healthy; who are you thinking of?
  b How old are they?
  c What makes you call them healthy? (open-ended)

Concept of health for self

Q.5 At times people are healthier than at other times. What is it like when *you* are healthy? (open-ended)

Ideas of cause – society at large

Q.3 a What do you think causes people to be healthier now than in your parents' time? (open-ended)
  b And what do you think causes people to be less healthy now than in your parents' time? (open-ended)

Ideas of cause – self

Q.17 Are there things about your life now that have a good effect on your health? What are they? (open-ended)

Q.18 Are there things about your health now that have a bad effect on your health? What are they? (open-ended)

Q.19 a Do you feel you lead a very healthy life/fairly healthy life/not very healthy life/unhealthy life?
  b What makes you say this? (open-ended)

Ideas of cause – diseases

Q.16 a–k What do you believe causes (stomach ulcers, chronic bronchitis, high blood pressure, obesity or being overweight, migraine, liver trouble, a stroke, lung cancer, heart trouble, severe depression, piles or haemorrhoids)? (open-ended)

Health as value

Q.14 b How far do you agree with the following statement:
To have good health is the most important thing in life (strongly agree/agree/all depends, don't know/disagree/strongly disagree)

Locus of health control

Q.14 Level of agreement on a 5-point scale, with 'don't know, it depends' occupying a middle position, with the statements:
  a It's sensible to do exactly what the doctors say
  c Generally health is a matter of luck
  d If you think too much about your health, you are more likely to be ill
  e Suffering sometimes has a divine purpose
  f I'd have to be very ill before I'll go to the doctor
  g People like me don't really have time to think about their health
  h The most important thing is the constitution you are born with

These statements were adapted from the literature on health locus of control (see e.g. Wallston and Wallston 1978) and the instrument was developed in the normal manner for a Likert scale. Agreement with statements c, e, g, h, was found to cluster with disagreement with statements a, d, f. Five categories were derived from the scores, with an approximately normal distribution.

Indices of the importance given to smoking, alcohol, diet, exercise

A score for each – arbitrarily divided into three categories of 'low', 'average' and 'high' – based on the number of times the behaviour was spontaneously mentioned in answers to attitudinal questions, i.e. Q. 3, 16, 17, 18, 19 above, and also

Q.7 b What are the three most important things you do to keep or improve your health? (open-ended)

Q.8 a Are there any things you would like to do to keep yourself healthy but don't?
  b What would you like to do? (open-ended)

Q.13 a Do you think it is ever people's own fault if they get ill? (open-ended)
  b (if yes) Why do you think it's their fault if they get ill? (open-ended)

REFERENCES

Ajzen, I. and Fishbein, N. (1980) *Understanding attitudes and predicting social behaviour*, Eaglewood Cliffs: Prentice Hall.

Anderson, R. (1983) 'How have people changed their health behaviour?', *Health Education Journal* 42: 82–86.

Anderson, R. (1984) 'Health promotion: an overview', *European Monographs on Health and Education Research* 6: 1–76.

Antonovsky, A. (1979) *Health, stress and coping. New perspectives on mental and physical well-being*, San Francisco: Jossey-Bass.

Antonovsky, A. (1984) 'The sense of coherence as a determinant of health', in J.P. Matarazzo (ed.) *Behavioural health*, New York: Wiley.

Arber, S. (1987) 'Social class, non-employment, and chronic illness: continuing the inequalities in health debate', *British Medical Journal* 294: 1069–73.

Arber, S., Gilbert, G.N., and Dale, A. (1985) 'Paid employment and women's health: a benefit or a source of role strain?' *Sociology of Health and Illness* 7: 375–400.

Ashley, F., Kanne, N., Sorlic, P., and Masson, R. (1975) 'Pulmonary function: relationship to ageing, cigarette habit and mortality', *Annals of Internal Medicine* 82: 739–45.

Balinsky, W. and Berger, R. (1975) 'A review of the research on general health status indexes', *Medical Care* 13: 283–318.

Banks, M.H. (1975) 'Factors influencing the demand for primary medical care in women aged 20–44 years', *International Journal of Epidemiology* 4: 189.

Banks, M.H. and Jackson, P.R. (1982) 'Unemployment and risk of minor psychiatric disorder in young people: cross-sectional and longitudinal evidence', *Psychological Medicine* 12: 789–798.

Beale, N. and Nethercott, S. (1985) 'Job loss and family morbidity: a study of a factory closure', *Journal of the Royal College of General Practitioners* 35; 510–14.

Becker, M.H. (ed.) (1974) 'The health belief model and personal health behaviour', *Health Education Monographs* 2; 326.

Belloc, N.B. (1973) 'Relationship of health practices and mortality', *Preventive Medicine* 2; 67–81.

Belloc, N.B. and Breslow, L. (1972) 'Relationship of physical health status and health practices', *Preventive Medicine* 1: 409–21.

Belloc, N.B., Breslow, L., and Hochstim, J.R. (1971) 'Measurement of physical health in a general population survey', *American Journal of Epidemiology* 93: 328–36.

Bergner, M., Bobbit, R.A., Kressel, S., Pollard, W.E., Gilson, B.S., and Morris, J.R. (1976) 'The sickness impact profile: conceptual formulation and methodology for the development of a health status measure', *International Journal of Health Services* 6: 393–415.

Berkman, L.F. and Breslow, L. (1983) *Health and ways of living: the Alameda County Study*, Oxford: Oxford University Press.

Berkman, L.F. and Syme S.L. (1979) 'Social networks, host resistance and mortality: a nine-year follow-up study of Alameda County residents', *American Journal of Epidemiology* 109: 186–204.

Blaxter, M. (1983) 'The causes of disease: women talking', *Social Science and Medicine* 17: 59–69

Blaxter, M. (1985) 'Self-definition of health status and consulting rates in primary care', *Quarterly Journal of Social Affairs* 1: 131–71.

Blaxter, M. (1987) 'Evidence on inequality in health from a national survey', *Lancet* i: 30–33, July.

Blaxter, M. (1989) 'A comparison of measures of morbidity', in J. Fox (ed.) *Health inequalities in European countries*, Aldershot: Gower Press.

Blaxter, M. and Paterson, E. (1982) *Mothers and daughters: a three-generational study of health attitudes and behaviour*, London: Heinemann Educational Books.

Boddy, F.A. and Forbes, J.F. (1981) *Small area variations in indices of maternal and child health: Glasgow 1975–77* Social Paediatric and Obstetric Research Unit, Glasgow.

Brenner, M.H. and Mooney, A. (1983) 'Unemployment and health', in M. Harrington (ed.) *Recent advances in occupational health*, Edinburgh: Churchill Livingstone.

Breslow, L. (1972) 'A quantitative approach to the World Health Organization definition of health: physical, social and mental well-being', *International Journal of Epidemiology* 1: 347.

Breslow, L. (1978) 'Prospects for improving health through reducing risk factors', *Preventive Medicine* 7: 449–58.

Breslow, L. and Enstrom J.E. (1980) 'Persistence of health habits and their relationship to mortality', *Preventive Medicine* 9: 469–83.

Brown, V.A. (1981) 'From sickness to health', *Social Science and Medicine* 15: 195–201.

Brown, G.W. and Harris, T. (1978) *Social origins of depression*, London: Tavistock.

Bryne, D., McCarthy P., Keighly J., and Harrison, S. (1985) 'Housing, class and health: an example of an attempt at doing socialist research', *Critical Social Policy* 13: 49–72.

Burr, M.L., St Leger, A.S., and Yarnell, J.W.G. (1981) 'Wheezing, dampness and coal fires', *Community Medicine* 3: 205–9.

Calnan, M. (1984) 'The Health Belief Model and participation in programmes for the early detection of breast cancer: a comparative analysis', *Social Science and Medicine* 19: 823–30.

Calnan, M. (1985) 'Patterns in preventive behaviour: a study of women in middle age', *Social Science and Medicine* 20: 263–8.

Calnan, M. (1987) *Health and illness*, London: Tavistock.

Calnan, M. and Johnson, B. (1985) 'Health, health risks and inequalities: an exploratory study of women's perceptions', *Sociology of Health and Illness* 7: 55–75.

Cameron, D. and Jones I.G. (1985) 'An epidemiological and sociological analysis of the use of alcohol, tobacco and other drugs of solace', *Community Medicine* 7: 18–24.

Carstairs, V. (1981) 'Small area analysis and health service research', *Community Medicine* 3: 131–9.

Cartwright, A. and Anderson, R. (1981) *General practice revisited*, London: Tavistock.

Cartwright, A., Hockey, L., and Anderson, J.L. (1973) *Life before death*, London: Routledge & Kegan Paul.

Cassel, J. (1976) 'The contribution of the social environment to host resistance', *American Journal of Epidemiology* 104: 107–23.

Chadwick, E. (1842) *Report to Her Majesty's Principal Secretary of State for the Home Department from the Poor Law Commissioners on an Enquiry into the Sanitary Condition of the Labouring Population of Great Britain*: M.W. Flinn (ed.) (1965), Edinburgh Press.

Chen, M.K. and Bryant, B.E. (1975) 'The measurement of health – a critical and selective overview', *International Journal of Epidemiology* 4: 257–64.

Cobb, S. (1976) 'Social support as a moderator of life stress', *Psychosomatic Medicine* 17: 405–11.

Cole-Hamilton, I. and Lang, T. (1986) *Tightening belts: a report on the impact of poverty on food*, London: London Food Commission.

Coleman, A. (1985) *Utopia on trial: vision and reality in planned housing*, London: Shipman.

Cook, D.G., Bartley, M.J., Cummins, R.O., and Shaper, A.G. (1982) 'Health of unemployed middle-aged men in Great Britain', *Lancet* i 1290–4.

Cook, D. and Shaper, A.G. (1984) 'Unemployment and health', in M. Harrington, (ed.) *Recent advances in occupational health*, Edinburgh: Churchill Livingstone.

Cornwell, J. (1984) *Hard-earned lives: accounts of health and illness from East London*, London: Tavistock Press.

Cox, B.D., Blaxter, M., Buckle, A.L.J., Fenner, N.P., Golding, J.F., Gore, M., Huppert, F.A. Nickson, J., Roth, Sir M., Stark, J., Wadsworth, M.E.J., and Whichelow, M. (1987) *The Health and Lifestyle Survey: preliminary report*, London: The Health Promotion Research Trust.

Craig, J. (1985) 'A 1981 socio-economic classification of local and health authorities of Great Britain', *Studies on Medical and Population Subjects* 48, Office of Population Censuses and Surveys, London: HMSO.

Crawford, R. (1984) 'A cultural account of "health": control, release and the social body', in J.B. McKinlay *Issues in the political economy of health care education*, New York: Tavistock Press.

CREDOC, (1982) *Morbidité et conditions de vie*, Paris.

Dean, K. (1984) 'Influence of health beliefs on lifestyles: what do we know?', *European Monographs in Health Education Research* 6: 127–49.

Dean, K. (1986) 'Social support and health: pathways of influence', *Health Promotion* 1: 133–50.

Department of Employment (annually) *Family Expenditure Survey*, London: HMSO.

Department of the Environment (1981) *An investigation of 'difficult to let' housing*, 3 volumes, London: HMSO.

Department of Health and Social Security (1976) *Prevention and health: everybody's business – a reassessment of public and personal health*, London HMSO.

Department of Health and Social Security (1980) *Inequalities in health* (The Black Report), London: HMSO.

Department of Health and Social Security (1981) *Care in action: a handbook of policies and priorities for the health and personal social services in England*, London: HMSO.

d'Houtard, A. and Field, M.G. (1984) 'The image of health: variations in perception by social class in a French population', *Sociology of Health and Illness* 6: 30–60.

Dight, S. (1976) *Scottish drinking habits*, Edinburgh: HMSO.

Dohrenwend, B.S. and Dohrenwend, B.P. (1974) *Stressful life events: their nature and effects*, New York: Wiley.

Dubos, R. (1961) *Mirage of health*, New York: Andor Books.

Dubos, R. (1971) *Man adapting*, New Haven: Yale University Press.

Elinson, J. (1974) 'Toward socio-medical health indicators', *Social Indicators Research* 1: 59–71.

Engel, G.L. (1977) 'The need for a new medical model: a challenge for biomedicine', *Science* 196: 129–36.

Fanshel, S. and Bush, J.W. (1970) 'A health-status index and its application to health-services outcomes', *Operations Research* 18: 1021–33.

Fisher, L.A. (1980) 'Effectiveness and efficiency in health education', Health Economics Research Unit discussion paper 09/80.

Fox, A.J. and Adelstein, A.M. (1978) 'Occupational mortality: work or way of life', *Journal of Epidemiology and Community Health* 32: 73–8.

Fox, A.J. and Goldblatt, P.O. (1982) *Longitudinal study: socio-demographic mortality differentials*. Series LS No. 1, OPCS, London HMSO.

Fox, A.J., Goldblatt, P.O., and Jones, D.R. (1986) 'Social class mortality differentials: artefact, selection, or life circumstances?', in

R.G. Wilkinson (ed.) *Class and health: research and longitudinal data*, London: Tavistock.

Fox, A.J., Jones, D.R., and Goldblatt, P.O. (1984) 'Approaches to studying the effect of socio-economic circumstances on geographic differences in mortality in England and Wales', *British Medical Bulletin* 40, 4: 309–14.

Garrad, J. and Bennett, A.E. (1971) 'A validated interview schedule for use in population surveys of chronic disability and disease', *British Journal of Preventive and Social Medicine* 25: 97–104.

Garrity, T.F., Somes, G.W. and Marx, M.B. (1978) 'Factors influencing self-assessments of health', *Social Science and Medicine* 12: 77–81.

Goldberg, D.P. (1972) *The detection of psychiatric illness by questionnaire*, London: Oxford University Press.

Goldberg, D. and Huxley, P. (1980) *Mental illness in the community*, London: Tavistock.

Graham, H. (1984) *Women, health and the family*, Brighton: Wheatsheaf Books.

Graham, H. (1986) *Caring for the family*, Research Report No. 1, London: Health Education Council.

Graham, H. (1987) 'Women's smoking and family health', *Social Science and Medicine* 25: 47–56.

Haavid-Mannila, E. (1986) 'Inequalities in health and gender', *Social Science and Medicine* 22: 141–9.

Haberman, P.W. (1969) 'The reliability and validity of the data', in J. Kosa, A. Antonovsky, and I. Zola (eds.) *Poverty and health*, Cambridge: Harvard University Press.

Hagart, J. and Billington, D.R. (1982) 'Towards an understanding of health status: the perceived importance of health status dimensions', *Community Medicine* 4: 12–24.

Hall, J. (1983) 'Subjective measures of quality of life in Britain: 1971–1975. Some developments and trends', *Social Trends* 7: 47–60.

Hannay, D.R. (1978) 'Symptom prevalence in the community', *Journal of the Royal College of General Practitioners* 28: 492–9.

Harris, D.M. and Guten, S. (1979) 'Health-protective behaviour: an exploratory study', *Journal of Health and Social Behaviour* 2, 17–29.

Hart, N. (1986) 'Inequalities in health: the individual versus the environment', *Journal of the Royal Statistical Society* A, 149: 228–46.

Hasan, J. (1986) 'The contribution of stress to differences in morbidity between occupational classes', paper presented to ESF Workshop on Inequality in Health, London (mimeo).

Hawton, K. and Rose, N. (1986) 'Unemployment and attempted suicide among men in Oxford', *Health Trends* 8: 29–32.

Headey, B., Homstrom, E. and Wearing, A. (1985) 'Models of well-being and ill-being', *Social Indicators Research* 17: 8–10.

Hellevik, O. (1984) *Introduction to causal analysis*, London: Allen & Unwin.

Herzlich, C. (1973) *Health and illness: a social psychological analysis*, London: Academic Press.

Holmes, T.H. and Rahe, R.H. (1967) 'The social maladjustment rating scale', *Journal of psychosomatic research* 11: 213–18.

House, J.A., Robbins, C., and Metzner, H.L. (1982) 'The association of social relationships and activities with mortality: prospective evidence from the Tecumseh Community Health Study', *American Journal of Epidemiology* 116: 123–40.

Hunt, S.M. (1986) 'Housing and health in a deprived area of Edinburgh', Conference of Institution of Environmental Health Officers, Warwick University (mimeo).

Hunt, S.M. and McEwen, J. (1980) 'The development of a subjective health indicator', *Sociology of Health and Illness* 2: 231–46.

Hunt, S.M., McKenna, S.P., McEwan, J., Backett, E.M., Williams, J., and Papp, E. (1980) 'A quantitative approach to perceived health status: a validation study', *Journal of Epidemiology and Community Health* 34: 281–6.

Illsley, R. (1986) 'Occupational class, selection and the production of inequalities in health,' *Quarterly Journal of Social Affairs* 2: 151–65.

Kantor, S. and Winkelstein, N. (1969) 'The rationale and use of ridit analysis in epidemiologic studies of blood pressure', *American Journal of Epidemiology* 90: 208.

Kaplan, R.M., Bush, J.W., and Barry, C.C. (1976) 'Health status: types of validity and the index of well-being', *Health Services Research* 11: 479–507.

Kaplan, G. and Cowles, A. (1978) 'Health locus of control and health value in the prediction of smoking reduction', *Health Education Monographs* 6: 129–37.

Kasl, S.V., Cobb, S., and Gore, S. (1972) 'Changes in reported illness and illness behaviour related to termination of employment', *International Journal of Epidemiology* 1: 111–18.

Katz, S., Ford, A.B., Moscowitz, R.W., Jackson, B.A., Jaffe, M.W., and Cleveland, M.A. (1963) 'Studies of illness in the aged. The index of ADL. A standardized measure of biological and psychosocial function', *Journal of American Medical Association* 185: 914–19.

Keithley, J., Byre, D., Harrison, S., and McCarthy P. (1984) 'Health and housing conditions in public sector housing estates', *Public Health* (London) 98: 344–53.

Kirshner, B. and Guyatt, G. (1985) 'A methodological framework for assessing health indices', *Journal of Chronic Diseases* 38: 27–36.

Kirscht, J.P. (1971) 'Social and psychological problems of surveys on health and illness', *Social Science and Medicine* 5: 519–26.

Koch, R. (1980) 'Verber bakteriologische Forschung', *Verhandlungen des X Internationalen Medizinischen Kongresses Berlin*, Berlin: Hirschwald.

Kohn, R. and White, K.L. (1976) *Health care: an international study*, Oxford: Oxford University Press.

Koskinen, S. (1985) 'Time trends in cause-specific mortality by occupational class in England and Wales IUSSP Conference, Florence.

Kreitman, N. and Platt, S. (1984) 'Suicide, unemployment and domestic

257

gas detoxification. *Journal of Epidemiology and Community Medicine* 38: 1–6.

Langlie, J.K. (1977) 'Social networks, health beliefs and preventive health behaviour', *Journal of Health and Social Behaviour* 18: 244–60.

Leon, D. and Wilkinson, R.G. (1986) 'Inequalities in prognosis: sociodemographic differences in cancer and heart disease survival', paper presented to European Science Foundation Workshop on Inequalities in Health, London.

Levenson, H.I. (1974) 'Activism and powerful others: distinctions within the concepts of internal – external control', *Journal of Personality Assessment* 38: 377–83.

Lindsey-Reid, E. and Osborn, R.W. (1980) 'Readiness for exercise adoption', *Social Science and Medicine* 14: 139–46.

Locker, D. (1981) *Symptoms and illness: the cognitive organization of disorder*, London: Tavistock.

Lundberg, O. (1986) 'Class and health: comparing Britain and Sweden', *Social Science and Medicine* 23: 511–17.

MAFF (annually) *Household food consumption and expenditure. Annual report of the National Food Survey Committee*, London: HMSO.

McCarthy, P. (1985) 'Respiratory conditions: effects of housing and other factors', *Journal of Epidemiology and Community Health* 39: 15–19.

MacFarlane, A. and Cole, T. (1985) 'From depression to recession – evidence about the effects of unemployment on mothers' and babies' health 1930s–1980s', in L. Durward, (ed.) *Born unequal: perspectives on pregnancy and childbearing in unemployed families*, London: Maternity Alliance.

MacFarlane, A. and Mugford, M. (1984) *Birth counts: statistics of pregnancy and childbirth*, London: HMSO.

Maclure, A. and Stewart, G.T. (1984) 'Admission of children to hospitals in Glasgow: relation to unemployment and other deprivation variables', *Lancet* ii: 682–5.

McQueen, D. (1988) 'Directions for research in health behaviour related to health promotion: a general overview', in R. Anderson, J. Davies, I. Kickbusch, D. McQueen, and R. Turner, (eds.) *Health behaviour research*, Oxford: Oxford University Press.

Marmot, M.G. (1978) 'Changing social class distribution of heart disease', *British Medical Journal* 2: 1109–12.

Marmot, M.G. (1986) Social inequalities in mortality: the social environment, in R.G. Wilkinson (ed.) *Class and health: research and longitudinal data*, London: Tavistock.

Marmot, M.G. and McDowall, M.E. (1986) 'Mortality decline and widening social inequalities', *Lancet* ii: 274–6.

Marmot, M.G., Rose, G., Shipley, M.J., and Hamilton, P.J.S. (1978) 'Employment grade and coronary heart disease in British civil servants', *Journal of Epidemiology and Community Health* 32: 244–9.

Marmot, M.G., Rose, G., Shipley, M.J., and Thomas, B.J. (1981) 'Alcohol and mortality: a U-shaped curve', *Lancet* i: 580.

Marmot, M.G., Shipley, M.J., and Rose, G. (1984) 'Inequalities in death-specific explanations of a general pattern?', *Lancet* i: 1003–6.

Marsh, A. (1985) 'Smoking and illness: what smokers really believe', *Health Trends* 17: 7–13.

Marsh, A. and Matheson, J. (1983) *Smoking attitudes and behaviour*, London: HMSO.

Mechanic, D. (1979) 'The stability of health and illness behaviour: results from a 16-year follow-up', *American Journal of Public Health* 69: 1142.

Mechanic, D., and Cleary, P.D. (1980) 'Factors associated with the maintenance of positive health behaviour', *Preventive Medicine* 9: 805.

Milne, J.S., Hope, K., and Williamson, J. (1970) 'Variability in replies to a questionnaire on symptoms of physical illness', *Journal of Chronic Disease* 22: 805–10.

Mishler, E.G. (1981) *Social contexts of health, illness and patient care*, Cambridge: Cambridge University Press.

Morris, J.N. (1983) 'Exercise, health and medicine', *British Medical Journal* 286: 1597–8.

Morris, J.N., Everitt, M.G., Pollard, R., Chave, S.P.W., and Semmence, A.M. (1980) 'Vigorous exercise in leisure-time: protection against coronary heart disease', *Lancet* ii: 1207–10.

Moser, K.A., Fox, A.J., and Jones, D.R. (1984) 'Unemployment and mortality in the OPCS longitudinal study', *Lancet* ii: 1324–9.

Moser, K.A., Fox, A.J., and Jones, D.R. (1986) 'Unemployment and mortality in the OPCS longitudinal study', in R.G. Wilkinson (ed.) *Class and health: research and longitudinal data*, London: Tavistock Press.

Moser, K.A. Fox, A.J., and Jones D.R. (1987) 'Unemployment and mortality: a comparison of the 1971 and 1981 longitudinal study census samples', *British Medical Journal* 294: 86–90.

Nathanson, C.A. (1978) 'Sex roles as variables in the interpretation of morbidity data', *International Journal of Epidemiology* 7: 253.

National Advisory Committee on Nutrition Education (1983) *Proposals for nutritional guidelines for health education in Britain*, London: Health Education Council.

National Center for Health Statistics (1964) *Health survey procedure: concepts, questionnaire development and definitions in the National Health Survey*, Series 1, No. 2, Public Health Service, Washington.

National Center for Health Statistics (1967) *US National Health Survey health interview responses compared with medical records. Vital and health statistics* 2, 23, Public Health Service, Washington.

O'Cummins, R., Shaper, A.G., Walker, M., and Wale C.J. (1981) 'Smoking and drinking by middle-aged British men: effects of social class and town of residence', *British Medical Journal* 283: 1497–1502.

Office of Population Censuses and Surveys (at intervals) *General Household Survey*, London: HMSO.

Office of Population Censuses and Surveys (1986) *Occupational mortality: decennial supplement 1979–80, 1982–83*, London: HMSO.

Pamuk, E.R. (1985) 'Social class inequality in mortality from 1921 to 1972 in England and Wales', *Population Studies* 39: 17–31.

Patrick, D.L., Darby, S.C., and Green, S.C. (1981) 'Screening for disability in the inner city', *Journal of Epidemiology and Community Health* 35: 65–70.

Pearlin, K. and Schooler, C. (1978) 'The structure of coping', *Journal of Health and Social Behaviour* 19: 2–21.

Pernanen, K. (1974) 'Validity of survey data on alcohol use', in *Research Advances in Alcohol and Drug Problems*, New York: Wiley.

Pill, R. and Stott, N.C.H. (1981) 'Relationship between health locus of control and belief in the relevance of lifestyle to health', *Patient Counselling and Health Education* 3: 95–9.

Pill, R. and Stott, N.C.H. (1982) 'Concept of illness causation and responsibility: some preliminary data from a sample of working class mothers', *Social Science and Medicine* 16: 43–52.

Pill, R. and Stott, N.C.H. (1985) 'Preventive procedures and practices among working class women: new data and fresh insights', *Social Science and Medicine* 21: 975–83.

Pill, R. and Stott, N.C.H. (1986) 'Looking after themselves: health protective behaviour among British working class women', *Health Education Research* 1: 111–19.

Platt, S. and Kreitman, N. (1984) 'Unemployment and parasuicide in Edinburgh 1968–82', *British Medical Journal* 289: 1029–32.

Rabkin, J.G. and Streuning E.L. (1976) 'Life events, stress and illness', *Nature* 194: 1013–20.

Reynolds, W.J., Rushing, W.A. and Miles, D.L. (1983) 'The validation of a function status index', *Journal of Health and Social Behaviour* 15: 271–83.

Richards, N.D. (1975) 'Methods and effectiveness of health education: the past, present and future of social scientific involvement', *Social Science and Medicine* 9: 141–56.

Rose, G. and Marmot, M. (1981) 'Social class and coronary heart disease', *British Heart Journal* 45: 13–19.

Rosenstock, I.M. (1969) 'Prevention of illness and maintenance of health', in J. Kosa, A. Antonovsky, and I.K. Zola, (eds.) *Poverty and health*, Cambridge: Harvard University Press.

Rosenstock, I.M. (1974) 'Historical origins of the health belief model', *Health Education Monographs* 2: 328–35.

Royal College of Physicians (1983) 'Obesity report', *Journal of the Royal College of Physicians* 17: 5–65.

Royal College of Psychiatrists (1978) *Alcohol and alcoholism*, London: Tavistock.

Ryle, J. (1961) 'The meaning of normal', in B. Lush, (ed.) *Concepts of medicine*, New York: Pergamon Press.

Sackett, D.L., Chambers, L.W., MacPherson, A.S., Goldsmith, C.H., and McAuley, R.G. (1977) 'The development and application of indices of health: general methods and a summary of results', *American Journal of Public Health* 67: 423–7.

Sainsbury, S. (1973) *Measuring disability*. Occasional papers on Social

Administration 54, the Social Administration Research Trust, London: G. Bell and Sons.

Sarason, I.G., Johnson, J.H., and Siegel, J.M. (1978) 'Assessing the impact of life changes: development of the life experiences survey', *Journal of Consulting and Clinical Psychology* 46: 932–46.

Scambler, A., Scambler, G., and Craig, D. (1981) 'Kinship and friendship networks and women's demand for primary care', *Journal of the Royal College of General Practitioners* 26: 746–50.

Scott Samuel, A. (1977) 'Social area analysis in community medicine', *British Journal of Preventive and Social Medicine* 31: 199–204.

Shaper, A.G., Pocock, S.J., Walker, M., Cohen, N.M., Wale, C.J., and Thomson, A.G. (1981) 'British regional heart study: cardiovascular risk factors in middle-aged men in 24 towns', *British Medical Journal* 283: 179–86.

Siegrist, J., Siegrist, K., and Weber, I. (1986) 'Sociological concepts of the etiology of chronic disease: the case of ischaemic heart disease', *Social Science and Medicine* 22: 247–53.

Singer, E., Garfinkel, R., Cohen, S.M., and Srole, L. (1976) 'Mortality and mental health: evidence from the Midtown Manhatten Restudy', *Social Science and Medicine* 10: 517.

Stacey, M. (1977) *Concepts of health and illness: a working paper on the concepts and their relevance for research*, London: Social Science Research Council.

Steele, J.L. and McBroom, W.H. (1972) 'Conceptual and empirical dimensions of health behaviour', *Journal of Health and Social Behaviour* 13: 382–92.

Stern, J. (1983a) 'Social mobility and the interpretation of social class mortality differentials', *Journal of Social Policy* 12: 27–49.

Stern, J. (1983b) 'The relationship between unemployment, morbidity and mortality in Britain', *Population Studies* 37: 61–74.

Sullivan, D.F. (1971) *Disability components for an index of health*, National Centre for Health Statistics, Vital and Health Statistics 2, 42, Washington: Public Health Service.

Syme, S.L. and Berkman, L.F. (1976) 'Social class susceptibility and sickness', *American Journal of Epidemiology* 104: 1–8.

Taylor, R. and Ford, G. (1981) 'Lifestyle and ageing: three traditions in lifestyle research', *Ageing and Society* 1: 329.

Theorell, T., Lind, E., and Floderus, B. (1975) 'The relationship of disturbing life-changes and emotions to the development of myocardial infarction and other serious illnesses', *International Journal of Epidemiology* 4: 281–93.

Thunhurst, C. (1985) *Poverty and health in the city of Sheffield*, Sheffield City Council Environmental Health Department.

Totman, R. (1979) *Social causes of illness*, London: Souvenir Press.

Townsend, P., Corrigan, P., and Kowarzik, O. (1986) *Poverty and the London labour market*, London: Low Pay Unit.

Townsend, P. and Davidson, N. (1982) *Inequalities in health: the Black Report*, Harmondsworth: Penguin Books.

Townsend, P., Phillimore, P., and Beattie, A. (1986) *Inequalities in health in the northern region: an interim report*, Northern Regional Health Authority/Bristol University.

Townsend, P., Simpson, D., and Tibbs, N. (1985) 'Inequalities in health in the city of Bristol; a preliminary review of statistical evidence', *International Journal of Health Services* 15: 637–63.

Unemployment and Health Study Group (1986) *Unemployment: a challenge to public health*, Centre for Professional Development, Dept. of Community Medicine, University of Manchester (mimeo).

Valkonen, T. (1987) *Social inequality in the face of death*, reprint 130, Dept. of Sociology, University of Helsinki.

Wadsworth, M.E.J. (1986) 'Serious illness in childhood and its association with later life achievement', in R.G. Wilkinson (ed.) *Class and health: research and longitudinal data*, London: Tavistock.

Waldron, I. (1983) 'Sex differences in illness incidence, prognosis and mortality: issues and evidence', *Social Science and Medicine* 17: 1107–23.

Wallston, K.A., Maides, S., and Wallston, B.S. (1976) 'Health-related information seeking as a function of health-related locus of control and health value', *Journal of Research in Personality* 10: 215–22.

Wallston, B.S. and Wallston K.A. (1978) 'Locus of control and health: a review of the literature', *Health Education Monographs* 6: 107–16.

Wallston, K.A., Wallston, B.S., and DeVellis, R. (1978) 'Development of the multi-dimensional health locus of control (MHLC) scales', *Health Education Monographs* 6: 160–70.

Wallston, B.S., Wallston, K.A., Kaplan, R.M., and Maides, S.A. (1976) 'Development and validation of the health locus of control (HLC) scale, *Journal of Consulting and Clinical Psychology* 44: 580–5.

Ware, J.E., Brook, R.H., Davies, A.R., and Lohr, K.N. (1981), 'Choosing measures of health status for individuals in general populations', *American Journal of Public Health* 71: 620–5.

Warr, P. (1984) 'Work and unemployment', in Drenth, P.J.D. *et al.* (eds.) *Handbook of work and organizational psychology*, London: John Wiley & Sons.

Warr, P. (1985) 'Twelve questions about unemployment and health', in Roberts, B., Finnegan, R., and Gallie, D. (eds.) *New approaches to economic life*, Manchester: Manchester University Press.

Webber, R. and Craig, J. (1978) 'Socio-economic classifications of Local Authority areas', *OPCS studies on medical and population subjects*, 35, London: HMSO.

Welin, L., Tibblin, G., Tibblin, B., Svardsudd, K., Ander-Peciva, S., Larrson, B., and Wilhelmsen, L. (1985) 'Prospective study of social influences on mortality', *Lancet* ii: 915–18.

Whichelow, M., Golding, J.F., and Treasure, S.P. (1988) 'A comparison of some dietary habits of smokers and non-smokers', *British Journal of Addiction* 83: 295–304.

Whitehead, M. (1987) *The health divide: inequalities in health in the 1980s*, London: Health Education Council.

Wiley, J.A. and Camacho, T.C. (1980) 'Lifestyle and future health: evidence from the Alameda County study', *Preventive Medicine* 9: 1–21.

Wilkinson, R.G. (1986a) 'Socio-economic differences in mortality: interpreting the data on their size and trends', in R.G. Wilkinson (ed.) *Class and health: research and longitudinal data*, London: Tavistock.

Wilkinson, R.G. (1986b) 'Income and mortality', in R.G. Wilkinson (ed.) *Class and health: research and longitudinal data*, London: Tavistock.

Wilkinson, R.G. (1986c) 'Occupational class, selection and inequalities in health; a reply to Raymond Illsley', *Quarterly Journal of Social Affairs* 2: 4.

Williams, R.G.A. (1979) 'Theories and measurement in disability', *Journal of Epidemiology and Community Health* 33: 32–47.

Williams, R.G.A. (1983) 'Concepts of health: an analysis of lay logic', *Sociology* 17: 185–204.

Wilson, P. (1980) *Drinking in England and Wales*, London: HMSO.

World Health Organization (1979) *Measurement of levels of health*, European series no. 7, Copenhagen: World Health Organization.

World Health Organization Regional Office for Europe (1984) *Health promotion: a discussion document on the concept and principles*, Copenhagen: World Health Organization.

World Health Organization (1985) *Targets for health for all, 2000*, Copenhagen: World Health Organization.

Wright, S. (1985) 'Subjective evaluation of health: a theoretical review', *Social Indicators Research 16*: 169–79.

Young, M. (1926) 'The variation in the mortality from cancer of different parts of the body in groups of men of different social status', *Journal of Hygiene* 25: 209–17.

INDEX